ABC OF ANTENATAL CARE

ABC OF
ANTENATAL CARE

GEOFFREY CHAMBERLAIN FRCOG

Professor and Chairman, Department of Obstetrics and Gynaecology,
St George's Hospital Medical School, London

Articles published in the *British Medical Journal*

Published by the British Medical Journal
Tavistock Square, London WC1H 9JR

First published 1992

British Library Cataloguing in Publication Data

Chamberlain, Geoffrey, 1930–
    ABC of antenatal care.
    618.24

ISBN 0–7279–0313–6

Front cover photograph: False colour, computer coded ultrasound image of fetus at 21 weeks. By courtesy of CNRI/ Science Photo Library.

Typesetting by Bedford Typesetters Ltd, Bedford
Printed in Great Britain at the University Press, Cambridge

Contents

	Page
Introduction	viii
Organisation of antenatal care	1
The changing body in pregnancy	5
Normal antenatal management	9
Checking for fetal wellbeing	15
Detection and management of congenital abnormalities	21
Work in pregnancy	27
Vaginal bleeding in early pregnancy	31
Medical problems in pregnancy—I	37
Medical problems in pregnancy—II	42
Abdominal pain in pregnancy	46
Raised blood pressure in pregnancy	51
Antepartum haemorrhage	56
Small for gestational age	61
Preterm labour	66
Multiple pregnancy	71
Vital statistics of birth	76
L'envoi	80
Index	81

INTRODUCTION

Antenatal care has evolved this century from a philanthropic service for mothers and their unborn babies to multiphasic screening. Much has been added in the past few years but a lack of analytical scrutiny has meant that little has been taken away. Healthy mothers and fetuses need little high technology care but some screening is desirable to allocate them with confidence to the healthy group of pregnant women. Women and fetuses at high risk need all the scientific help available to ensure the safest environment for delivery and aftercare. The detection and successful management of women and fetuses at high risk are the science of antenatal care; the care of the other mothers at lower risk is the art of the subject and probably can proceed without much science. Midwives must be recognised as practitioners of normal obstetrics, and they will in the future take over much of the care of the normal pregnancies, backed up by general practitioner obstetricians in the community and by consultant led obstetrical teams in hospitals.

This book has evolved from over 30 years of practice, reading, and research. I have tried to unwind the tangled skeins of aetiology and cause, of rational and traditional management, but naturally what remains is an opinion. To broaden this I have sought advice from many friends, whom I thank. Specifically I thank Mr Malcolm Pearce and Dr Jennifer Davies of St George's Hospital for willingly giving good advice and not objecting when I did not follow all of it. Furthermore, many people have written to me after having read the individual articles in the *BMJ*; though only a few letters were published, I have benefited from many freely given comments and have incorporated them in this book. Finally, I am indebted to Mr Andrew Rolland, photographer, to Dr Rashmi Patel, ultrasonologist, to Mrs Anne Fraser, my secretary, and to Ms Sharon Davies, my technical editor at the *BMJ*.

GEOFFREY CHAMBERLAIN

Professor of Obstetrics,
St George's Hospital,
London
August 1991

ORGANISATION OF ANTENATAL CARE

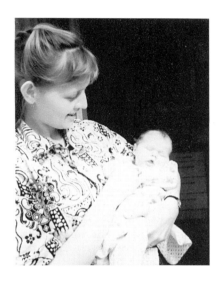

Looking after pregnant women presents one of the paradoxes of modern medicine. Normal women proceeding through an uneventful pregnancy require little formal medicine. Conversely, those at high risk of damage to their own health or that of their fetus require the use of appropriate scientific technology. Accordingly, there are two classes of women, the larger requiring support but not much intervention and the other needing the full range of diagnostic and therapeutic measures as in any other branch of medicine. To distinguish between the two is the aim of well run antenatal care.

Antenatal clinics provide a multiphasic screening service; the earlier that women are screened to identify those at high risk of specified problems the sooner appropriate diagnostic tests can be used to assess such women and their fetuses and treatment can be started. As always in medicine, diagnosis must precede treatment, for unless the women who require treatment can be identified specifically, management cannot be correctly applied.

Background

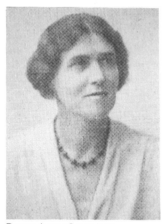

Dame Janet Campbell.

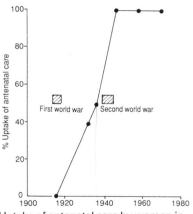

Uptake of antenatal care by women in England and Wales.

Women attend for antenatal care because they expect it. They have been brought up to believe that antenatal care is the best way of looking after themselves and their unborn children. This is reinforced in all educational sources from medical textbooks to women's magazines.

Prenatal care started in Edinburgh at the turn of the century, but clinics for the checking of apparently well pregnant women were rare before the first world war. During the 1920s a few midwifery departments of hospitals and interested general practitioners saw women at intervals to check their urine for protein. Some palpated the abdomen, but most pregnant women had only a medical or midwifery consultation once before labour, when they booked. Otherwise, doctors were concerned with antenatal care only "if any of the complications of pregnancy should be noticed." Obstetrics and midwifery were first aid services concerned with labour and its complications: virtually all vigilance, thought, and attention centred on delivery and its mechanical enhancement. Little attention was paid to the antenatal months.

During the 1920s a wider recognition emerged of the maternal problems of pregnancy as well as those of labour; the medical profession and the then Ministry of Health woke up to realise that events of labour had their precursors in pregnancy. Janet Campbell, one of the most farsighted and clear thinking women in medicine, started a national system of antenatal clinics with a uniform pattern of visits and procedures; her scheme of management can still be recognised today in all the clinics of the Western world.

Campbell's ideas became the clinical obstetric screening service of the 1930s. To it has been added a series of tests, often with more enthusiasm than scientific justification; over the years few investigations have been taken away, merely more added. Catalysed by the National Perinatal Epidemiological Unit in Oxford, various groups of more thoughtful obstetricians are now trying to sort out which of the tests are in fact useful in predicting fetal and maternal hazard and which have a low return for effort.

Organisation of antenatal care

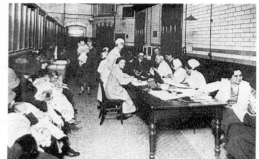

Antenatal clinics evolved from child welfare clinics, producing a prenatal version of the infant clinics.

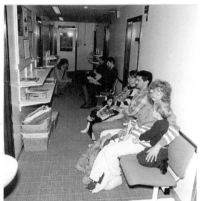

An antenatal clinic in the 1990s.

When this has been done a rational antenatal service may be developed, but until then we must work with a confused service that "growed like Topsy". It is a mixture of the traditional clinical laying on of hands and a patchily applied provision of complex tests, whose availability often depends as much on the whims of a health authority's ideas of priority as on the needs of the women and their fetuses.

As well as these economic considerations, doctors planning the care of women in pregnancy should consider the women's own wishes. Too often antenatal clinics have been designated cattle markets; the wishes of women coming for care should be sought and paid attention to. A recurrent problem is the apparent rush of the hospital clinic and the impersonal nature of care given by several different junior doctors and midwives, none of whom knows the woman well. The waiting time is a source of harassment and so is the time taken to travel to the clinic. Most women want time and a rapport with the antenatal doctor or midwife to ask questions and have them answered in a fashion they can understand. It is here that the midwife comes into her own for she is excellent at the care of women undergoing normal pregnancies.

In many parts of the country midwives run their own clinics in places where women go as part of daily life — for example, shopping centres. Here, midwives see a group of healthy normal women through pregnancy with two visits only to the hospital antenatal clinic. To get the best results women at higher risk need to be screened out at or soon after booking. Those at highest risk receive intensive care at the hospital consultant clinic and those at intermediary risk have shared care between the general practitioner and the hospital, while the women at lower risk are seen by the midwives at the community clinics. Programmes of this nature now run, many of them in Scotland. Janet Campbell started something in 1920. We should not necessarily think that the pattern she derived is right forever, and in the 1990s we may start to get it right for the current generation of women.

Styles of antenatal care

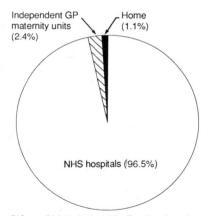

Place of birth in 1988 in England and Wales.

Claims by general practitioners for intranatal maternity services

	% Of births
Total claims for intranatal care	11·0
In independent GP units	2·5
At home	1·0
In combined GP and consultant NHS units	7·5

The type of antenatal care that a woman and her general practitioner elect will vary with local arrangements. The important first decision on which antenatal care plans depend is where the baby will be delivered. Ninety nine per cent of babies in the United Kingdom are now delivered in institutions; a half of the 1% of domiciliary deliveries are unplanned, so about 0·5% are booked as home deliveries. If the delivery is to be in an institution there is still the choice in some areas of general practitioner deliveries either at a separate unit run by general practitioners isolated from the hospital or in a combined unit with a consultant. Most deliveries take place in an NHS hospital under the care of a consultant team. A small but possibly increasing number in the next few years may be in private care, by a general practitioner obstetrician, a consultant obstetrician, or an independent midwife.

Once the plans for delivery are decided, the pattern of antenatal visits can be worked out. If the general practitioner is going to look after delivery antenatal care might be entirely in his hands, with the use of the local obstetric unit for investigations and consultation. At the other end of the spectrum, antenatal care is entirely in the hands of the hospital unit under a consultant obstetrician and a team of doctors and midwives, the general practitioner seeing nothing of the woman until she has been discharged from hospital after delivery.

Most women, however, elect for antenatal care between these two extremes. They often wish to take a bigger part in their own care. In some antenatal clinics the checking of weight and the dipstick test for proteinuria are done by the woman herself. As well as providing some satisfaction, this reduces the load and waiting time at the formal antenatal visit.

During pregnancy there are visits at certain agreed stages of gestation to

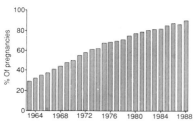

Claims by general practitioners for antenatal and postnatal care as a percentage of all pregnancies for which a claim was made.

the hospital antenatal clinic for crucial checks and for the rest of the time antenatal care is performed in the general practitioner's surgery. Here it may be by the practitioner or by a community midwife attached to the practice. These patterns of care keep the practitioner involved in the obstetric care of the woman and allow the woman to be seen in slightly more familiar surroundings. In some areas clinics outside the hospital are run by community midwives; these are becoming increasingly popular.

Delivery may be in the hospital by the consultant led team, by a general practitioner obstetrician, or by a midwife. It is wise, with the introduction of crown indemnity, that all general practitioner obstetricians have honorary contracts with the hospital obstetric department they attend to supervise or perform deliveries.

Diagnosis of pregnancy

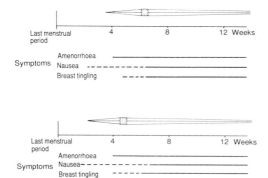

Time at which a group of primiparous (above) and multiparous women (below) first thought that they were pregnant in relation to the more conventional symptoms. The mean (box) and range are given in weeks of gestation.

When a woman attends a practitioner thinking that she is pregnant the most common symptoms are not always amenorrhoea followed by nausea. Many women have a subtle sensation that they are pregnant a lot earlier than the arrival of the more formal symptoms and signs laid down in textbooks. Traditionally, the doctor may elicit clinical features, but most now turn to a pregnancy test at the first hint of pregnancy.

Symptoms

The symptoms of early pregnancy are nausea, irritation of the breasts, increased frequency of micturition, and amenorrhoea.

Signs

The doctor may notice on examination a fullness of the breasts with early changes in pigmentation and Montgomery's tubercles in the areola. The uterus will not be felt through the abdominal wall until after 12 weeks of pregnancy. On bimanual assessment uterine enlargement is detectable before this time whereas cervical softening and a cystic, soft general feeling of the uterus can be detected by eight weeks. This more subtle sign is not often sought in the general practitioner's surgery as vaginal examination is not often performed.

Tests

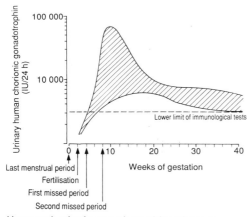

Human chorionic gonadotrophin values rise sharply in early gestation but are reduced in the second half of pregnancy. The range (2SD) are shown.

Mostly the diagnosis of pregnancy is confirmed by tests checking for the high concentrations of human chorionic gonadotrophin that occur in every pregnancy. The old biological tests using rabbits and frogs are now gone and have been replaced by immunological tests. These depend on the presence of human chorionic gonadotrophin in the body fluids, principally the urine. The more sensitive the test, the more likely it is to pick up the hormone at lower concentrations—that is, earlier in pregnancy. Also important, the test should be specific for human chorionic gonadotrophin so that it does not cross react with the pituitary gonadotrophins (follicle stimulating hormone and luteinising hormone), which are often present in increased concentrations in later reproductive life as the body tries to stimulate ovulation from an aging ovary.

Human chorionic gonadotrophin consists of two subunits—α and β. The α subunit is similar to that of the other gonadotrophins but the β subunit is specific to human chorionic gonadotrophin. Antibodies can be generated to the β subunit alone to increase the specificity of the tests. Furthermore, monoclonal antibodies prepared artificially enable these specific antibodies to the β subunit to be produced cheaply, thus permitting wider usage of these tests.

In practice the reaction of human chorionic gonadotrophin antigen with its antibody is made visible by attaching either the antigen or the antibody to latex particles. When both are present agglutination occurs, the particles adhering to each other and forming precipitates. Usually the antibody is coated on to the particles so that if precipitation occurs human chorionic gonadotrophin must have been present in the fluids to which it was added.

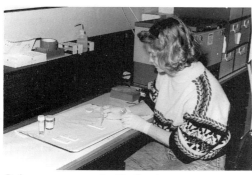

Doing a pregnancy test is simple.

3

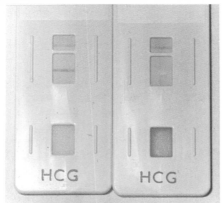

Clearview pregnancy test results. The horizontal bar in the top chamber shows that a urine sample has progressed satisfactorily from the lower chamber. A horizontal bar in the middle chamber shows a positive result (left) and its absence a negative result (right).

Enzyme linked immunosorbant assay (ELISA) is the basis of many of the commercial kits currently available in chemist shops. The assay depends on the double reaction of standard phase antibody with enzyme labelled antibody, which is sensitive and so able to detect very low concentrations of human chorionic gonadotrophin. Positive results are therefore detectable as early as 10 days after fertilisation—that is, four days before the first missed period.

Conclusions

Antenatal care has evolved from a hospital based to a community based service for normal women. Those with a higher risk of problems are best seen in hospital clinics.

At the end of the preliminary consultation women may ask questions about the pregnancy, and the practitioner will deal with these. Most of these queries will be considered in the chapter on normal antenatal management. For most women the onset of pregnancy is a desired and happy event, but for a few it may not be so and the practitioner, having established a diagnosis, may find that he is then asked to advise on termination of pregnancy. This he should do if his views on the subject allow; if not, he should arrange for one of his partners to discuss it with the woman. Most women, however, want the pregnancy, and it will continue to produce eventually a much desired result.

The picture of the infant welfare clinic is reproduced by permission of William Heinemann from *University College Hospital and its Medical School: a History* by W R Merrington. The Clearview pregnancy test result is reproduced by permission of Unipath, Bedford.

Recommended reading
Hall MH, ed. Antenatal care. *Baillieres Clin Obstet Gynaecol* 1990;4(1):1-233.

THE CHANGING BODY IN PREGNANCY

Pregnancy causes physiological and psychological changes, which all affect the woman's life

Pregnancy is a load causing alterations not just in the mother's pelvic organs but all over the woman's body. The fetus's physiology is different from that of an adult, but it interacts with the mother's systems, causing adaptation and change of function in her body. These adaptations generally move to minimise the stresses imposed and to provide the best environment for the growing fetus; they are usually interlinked smoothly so that the effects on the function of the whole organism are minimised. The changes will be dealt with briefly in this chapter.

Cardiovascular system

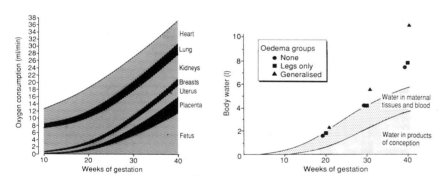

Increase in oxygen consumption (left) and body water (right) during pregnancy. A major part of the increase goes to the products of conception (fetus, placenta, and membranes).

The increased load on the heart in pregnancy is due to greater needs for oxygen in the tissues.

● The fetus's body and organs grow rapidly and its tissues have an even higher oxygen consumption per unit volume than the mother's

● The hypertrophy of most maternal tissues, not just the breast and uterus, increases oxygen requirements

● The mother's muscular work is increased to move her increased size and that of the fetus.

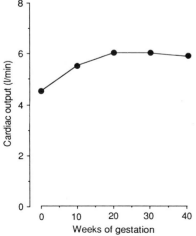

Cardiac output in pregnancy. The increase occurs very early and flattens from 20 weeks.

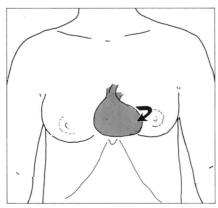

The heart becomes larger and rotates in a clockwise fashion (seen from above), unwinding on the roots of the great vessels.

Cardiac output is the product of stroke volume and heart rate. It is increased in pregnancy by a rise in pulse rate with a small increase in stroke volume. Cardiac muscle hypertrophy occurs so that the heart chambers enlarge and output increases by 40%; this occurs rapidly in the first half of pregnancy and steadies off in the second. In the second stage of labour cardiac output is further increased, with uterine effort increasing output by a further 30% at the height of the mother's pushing.

During pregnancy the heart is enlarged and pushed up by the growing mass under the diaphragm. The aorta is unfolded and so the heart is rotated upwards and outwards. This produces electrocardiographic and radiographic changes, which, although normal for pregnancy, may be interpreted as abnormal if a cardiologist or radiologist did not know of the pregnancy.

The changing body in pregnancy

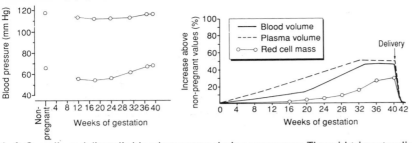

Left: Systolic and diastolic blood pressures during pregnancy. The mid-trimester dip found in some women is seen more in the diastolic than in the systolic pressure.
Right: Increase in blood volume and its components in pregnancy.

Blood pressure may be reduced in mid-pregnancy, but pulse pressure is increased and peripheral resistance generally decreased during pregnancy.

Maternal blood volume increases, the changes in plasma volume being proportionally greater than the increase in red cell bulk. Hence haemodilution occurs; this used to be called a physiological anaemia, a bad phrase as it is paradoxical to have a physiological pathological process.

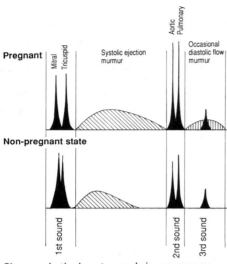

Changes in the heart sounds in pregnancy.

The heart sounds are changed:

● A systolic ejection murmur is common
● A third cardiac sound is commonly heard accompanying ventricular filling

The electrical activity of the heart on an electrocardiogram changes.

● The ventricles become hypertrophied, the left to a greater extent than the right and therefore left ventricular preponderance is seen in the QRS deviation
● The unfolding of the heart on the aortic and pulmonary tract may result in inverted T waves in V2 and sometimes V3 and in ST segment changes.

Changes in chest radiographs in pregnancy

Heart

● More horizontal so cardiothoracic ratio is increased
● Has a straighter left upper border

Lungs

● Show increased vascular soft tissue
● Often have a small pleural effusion especially straight after delivery

---

Heart valves and chamber volumes may change during pregnancy. These changes can be visualised by cross sectional echocardiography, which depends on the reflection of high frequency sound from inside the heart.

The most common changes seen on chest x ray films are shown in the box. Always ensure that the radiology department is told on the request form that a woman is pregnant and give an approximate stage of gestation. Only when there are strong indications should radiography be performed in pregnancy at all.

Respiratory system

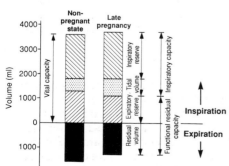

Changes in inspiratory and expiratory volumes in pregnancy.

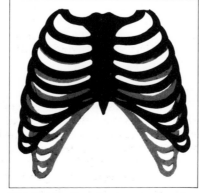

The rib cage is pushed upwards and outwards as pregnancy advances.

In early pregnancy women breathe more deeply but not more frequently under the influence of progesterone. Hence alveolar ventilation is increased by as much as a half above prepregnant values.

Later the growing uterus increases intra-abdominal pressure so that the lower ribs flare out and the diaphragm is pushed up. Expiratory reserve volume is decreased but the vital capacity is maintained by a slight increase in inspiratory capacity because of an enlarged tidal volume.

Urinary system

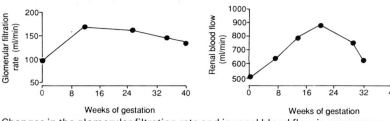

Changes in the glomerular filtration rate and in renal blood flow in pregnancy.

Changes in clearance
Renal blood flow is increased during early pregnancy by 40%. The increase in glomerular filtration rate (by 40%) is accompanied by enhanced tubular reabsorption; plasma concentrations of urea and creatinine decrease.

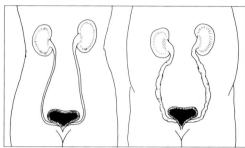

Changes in the ureters in pregnancy, during which they lengthen and become more tortuous and dilated.

The muscle of the bladder is relaxed because of increased circulating progesterone concentrations. Increased frequency of micturition due to increased urine production is a feature of early pregnancy. Later the organ is mechanically pressed on by the growing uterus and the same symptoms occur but for a different reason.

The muscle walls of the ureters are relaxed by progesterone so that the ureters become larger, wider, and of lower tone. Sometimes stasis occurs in the ureters; therefore proliferation of bacteria and the development of urinary infection is more likely to occur.

Endocrine system

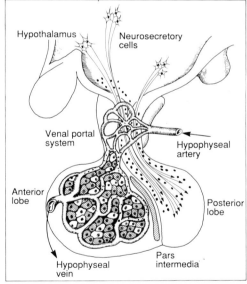

Pituitary gland showing secreting areas.

All the maternal endocrine organs are altered in pregnancy, largely because of the increased secretion of trophic hormones from the pituitary gland and the placenta.

Pituitary gland
The pituitary gland is increased in size during pregnancy, mostly because of changes in the anterior lobe.

- *Anterior lobe*
Prolactin—Within a few days of conception the rate of prolactin production increases. Concentrations rise until term following the direct stimulation of the lactotrophs by oestrogens. Human placental lactogen, which shows shared biological activity, exerts an inhibitory feedback effect. Prolactin affects water transfer across the placenta and therefore fetal electrolyte and water balance. It is later concerned with the production of milk, both initiating and maintaining milk secretion.
Gonadotrophins—The secretions of both follicular stimulating hormone and luteinising hormone are inhibited during pregnancy.
Growth hormone—The secretion of growth hormone is inhibited during pregnancy, probably by human placental lactogen. Metabolism in the acidophil cells returns to normal within a few weeks after delivery and is unaffected by lactation.
Adrenocorticotrophic hormone concentration increases slightly in pregnancy despite the rise in cortisol concentrations. The normal feedback mechanism seems to be inhibited secondary to a rise in binding globulin concentrations.
Thyrotrophin secretion seems to be the same as that in non-pregnant women. The main changes in thyroid activity in pregnancy come from non-pituitary influences.

- *Posterior lobe*
There are increases in the release of hormones from the posterior pituitary gland at various times during pregnancy and lactation. These, however, are produced in the hypothalamus, carried to the pituitary gland in the portal venous system, and stored there. The most important is oxytocin, which is released in spurts from the pituitary gland during labour to stimulate uterine contractions. Its secretion may also be stimulated by stretching of the lower genital tract. Oxytocin is also released during suckling and is an important part of the let down reflex.

Changes in prolactin concentrations in pregnancy (means (SEM)).

The changing body in pregnancy

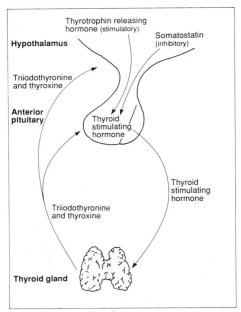

Control of thyroxine secretion in pregnancy.

Thyroid gland

Pregnancy is a hyperdynamic state and so the clinical features of hyperthyroidism may sometimes be seen. The basal metabolic rate is raised and the concentrations of thyroid hormone in the blood are increased, but thyroid function is essentially normal in pregnancy.

In pregnancy the renal clearance of iodine is greatly increased but thyroid clearance also rises so absolute iodine intake remains in the normal range.

Adrenal gland

The adrenal cortex synthesises cortisol from acetate or cholesterol. In pregnancy there is an increase in adrenocorticotrophic hormone concentration along with an increase in total plasma cortisol concentration because of raised binding globulin concentrations. The cortex also secretes an increased amount of renin, possibly because of the increased oestrogen concentrations. This enzyme produces angiotensin I, which is associated with maintaining blood pressure. Some renin also comes from the uterus and the chorion, which together produce a large increase in renin concentrations in the first 12 weeks of gestation. There is little change in deoxycorticosterone concentrations despite the swings in electrolyte balance in pregnancy.

The adrenal medulla secretes adrenaline and noradrenaline. The metabolism seems to be the same during pregnancy as before; the concentrations of both hormones rise in labour.

Placenta

The oestrogen, progesterone, and cortisol endocrine functions of the placenta are well known. In addition, many other hormones are produced with functions related to maternal adaptation to the changes of fetal growth.

Genital tract

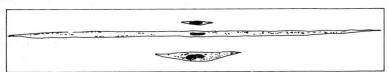

Myometrial cells from a non-pregnant uterus (top), a uterus in pregnancy (middle), and a uterus after pregnancy (bottom). The cells hypertrophy in length up to 20 times in pregnancy. After pregnancy they never quite return to their former size.

The uterus changes in pregnancy; the increase in bulk is due mainly to hypertrophy of the myometrial cells, which do not increase much in number but grow much larger. Oestrogens stimulate growth, and the stretching caused by the growing fetus and the volume of liquor provides an added stimulus to hypertrophy.

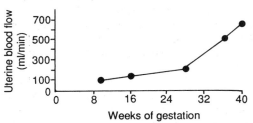

Changes in uterine blood flow in pregnancy.

The blood supply through the uterine and ovarian arteries is greatly increased so that at term 1·0-1·5 l of blood are perfused every minute. The placental site has a preferential blood supply, about 85% of the total uterine blood flow going to the placental bed.

The cervix, which is made mostly of connective tissue, becomes softer after the effect of oestrogen on the ground substance of connective tissue encourages an accumulation of water. The ligaments supporting the uterus are similarly stretched and thickened.

The figures showing the changes in heart sounds and murmurs during pregnancy and the control of thyroid secretion are reproduced by permission of Blackwell Scientific Publications from *Clinical Physiology in Obstetrics* edited by F Hytten and G Chamberlain. The figure showing prolactin secretion during pregnancy is reproduced by permission of the *American Journal of Obstetrics and Gynecology* (Rigg LA, Lein A, Yen SCC, 1977;**129**:454-6).

Recommended reading

Hytten F, Chamberlain G, eds. *Clinical physiology in obstetrics*. 2nd ed. Oxford: Blackwell Scientific Publications, 1990.

NORMAL ANTENATAL MANAGEMENT

Aims of antenatal care
- Management of maternal symptomatic problems
- Management of fetal symptomatic problems
- Screening and prevention of maternal problems
- Screening and prevention of fetal problems
- Preparation of the couple for childbirth
- Preparation of the couple for childrearing

Antenatal care in the 1990s has six functions (box). The first two are the same as any performed in an outpatient clinic (treatment of symptoms); the second two relate to multiphasic screening, of which antenatal care was an early example; the third pair are part of health education.

Antenatal care in the United Kingdom is performed by a range of professionals—midwives, general practitioners, and hospital doctors. In many areas up to 70% of antenatal care is in the hands of general practitioners and community midwives. In many parts of the country midwives hold their own clinics outside the hospital.

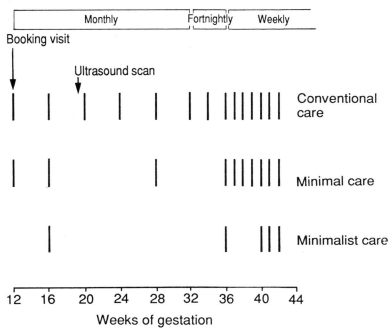

Intervals of antenatal visits: conventional pattern (top); current ideas of low risk care (middle); plan for the least number of visits (bottom).

In the United Kingdom many women book for antenatal care by 14 weeks and are seen at intervals. There is no association between the number of visits and outcome; in Switzerland there are an average of five and in The Netherlands as many as 14. The number of visits depends on a traditional pattern laid down by Dame Janet Campbell in the 1920s (see chapter on organisation of antenatal care) rather than on being planned with thoughts relating to the contemporary scene. A more rational plan of care of normal primigravidas and multigravidas is laid down by Dr Marion Hall of Aberdeen (tables). With these criteria, antenatal care would be more cost effective and no less clinically useful. When pioneers have tried to reduce the number of visits from the traditional number, however, there has been resistance from older obstetricians, conventional midwives, women having babies, and their mothers, all of whom think that Campbell's by now traditional pattern must be right.

As well as the clinical regimen, antenatal care now entails a whole series of complex tests, many of which have been added without proper assessment. They too have their correct times for application.

Minimum care for normal multigravidas

Week of gestation	Main purpose of visit*
12	History and examination, clarification of uncertain gestation, identification of risk factors for antenatal care and confinement, booking blood tests
	Advice on diet, drugs, work, and exercise
18-20	α Fetoprotein screening or ultrasound scan, or both
22	Fundal height, baseline weight
30	Fundal height, weight gain, identification of high risk of intrauterine growth retardation and pre-eclampsia
36	Fundal height, weight gain, identification of malpresentation
40	Assessment of need for induction

*Blood pressure reading and urine analysis are performed at every visit.

Visits for normal primigravidas in addition to minimum care for multigravidas

Week of gestation	Main purpose of visit
26	Blood pressure, urine analysis, discussion of delivery and feeding
34	Blood pressure, urine analysis, discussion of delivery and feeding
38	Blood pressure, urine analysis, discussion of delivery and feeding
41	Blood pressure, urine analysis, discussion of delivery and feeding

Prepregnancy care

Aims of prepregnancy care

- To bring the woman and her partner to pregnancy in the best possible health

- To provide the means of ensuring that preventable factors are attended to before pregnancy starts—for example, rubella inoculation

- To give advice about the effects of:
    - —pre-existing disease and its treatment on the pregnancy and unborn child
    - —the pregnancy on pre-existing disease and its treatment

- To consider the likelihood and effects of any recurrence of events from previous pregnancies or deliveries

---

Some aspects of a couple's way of life may be checked before pregnancy. The man and the woman's medical and social history, and, if relevant, her obstetric career can be assessed. Immunity from infections such as rubella can be tested; alternative treatments to some longstanding conditions such as ulcerative colitis can be discussed. The possibility of a recurrence of pre-existing problems such as deep vein thrombosis can be assessed. Dietary habits and problems at work can be assessed and changes in consumption of cigarettes or alcohol may be considered. Once pregnancy has started the couple have only one option—that is, to continue or stop the pregnancy. Prepregnancy care allows more time for the correction of detectable problems and the prevention of their repetition— for example, giving supplementary folate to women whose children have abnormalities of the central nervous system.

Booking visit

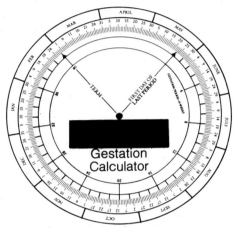

An adjustable obstetric calculator should always be used to calculate the current stage of gestation and the expected date of delivery.

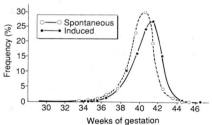

Distribution of length of gestation for spontaneous and induced single births when the last menstrual period is known (n=16 000).

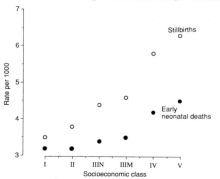

Stillbirths (per 1000 total births) and neonatal deaths in the first week (per 1000 live births) by socioeconomic class.

Once pregnancy has been diagnosed by the general practitioner the woman usually attends a booking visit at the clinic that she will go to for antenatal care. This is the longest but the most important visit. It used to take place at 8-12 weeks' gestation, but in many clinics it has moved into the middle trimester. The woman's medical state is assessed so that the current pregnancy can be placed into the appropriate part of a risk spectrum. Baseline data are essential at this point and are obtained from the history, an examination, and relevant investigations.

History

Symptoms that have arisen in the current pregnancy before the booking visit are ascertained—for example, vaginal bleeding and low abdominal pain.

Menstrual history—To assess the expected date of delivery details are needed about the last normal menstrual period including its date, the degree of certainty of that date, and whether cycles are reasonably regular around 28 days. The use of oral contraception or ovulation induction agents that might inhibit or stimulate ovulation should be discussed. A firm date for the last menstrual period can be obtained from about 80% of women at a British booking clinic. From this the expected date of delivery can be calculated with a calculator. Do not do sums in the head; they run into trouble when a pregnancy runs over the end of a year. A woman can be told that she has an 85% chance of delivering within a week of the expected date of delivery, but the general practitioner obstetrician would do well to emphasise at this point that this date is only a calculation of mathematical probability and, as with other odds, the favourite does not always win the race.

Medical history—Specific illnesses and operations of the past should be inquired about, particularly those that entail treatment that needs to be continued in pregnancy—for example, epilepsy and diabetes.

Family history—There may be conditions among first degree relatives (parents or siblings) that may be reflected in the current pregnancy, such as diabetes or twinning.

Sociobiological background—Age, parity, social class, and race of the woman all affect the outcome of the pregnancy. Smoking and alcohol consumption also take their toll. Socioeconomic class is usually derived from the occupation of the woman or her partner. It reflects the influence of a mixed group of factors such as nutrition in early life, diseases in childhood, education, and past medical care. It also correlates with potential birth weight, congenital abnormality rates, and eventually perinatal mortality.

Proportions of women in each socioeconomic class in England and Wales adjusted by job description of husband or partner

Social class	Job description	% Population having babies
I	Professional and managerial	6·3
II	Supervisory	18·8
III	Skilled	38·1
IV	Semiskilled	12·0
V	Unskilled	4·6
Not classifiable	Students / Armed forces / Unemployed*	10·9

*In many surveys unemployed people are classified by their last occupation if they had one.

Obstetric history—The woman's obstetric history should be gone into carefully as it contains some of the best markers for performance in the current pregnancy. If the woman has had a previous miscarriage or termination of pregnancy the doctor should ask about the stage of gestation, the degree of certainty of the pregnancy, and any illness afterwards. Of babies born, the progress of the pregnancy, labour, and puerperium are needed and the stage of gestation and birth weight of the infant. Intrauterine growth retardation and preterm labour may be recurrent and should be inquired about in previous pregnancies. The terms gravidity and parity are often applied to women in pregnancy. Gravidity is the Latin word for pregnancy, so anyone who is gravid is or has been pregnant. A woman who is pregnant for the first time is a primigravida. Parity refers to having given birth in the past to an infant—that is, a liveborn or a stillborn child.

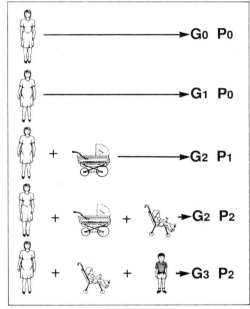

Gravity (G) and parity (P).

Examination

A brief but relevant physical examination should be performed. The woman's height is important as it correlates loosely with pelvic size, but shoe size is a poorer predictor. Taking her weight is useful as a baseline reading to be able to assess weight gain later in pregnancy. The clinical presence of anaemia should be checked and a brief examination of the teeth included, if only to warn the woman to go to see a dentist. Tooth and gum deterioration may be rapid in pregnancy and dental care is free at this time and for a year after delivery. Check whether the thyroid gland is enlarged. The heart and lungs are auscultated for gross disorders, although most major problems will be known to the woman and have been discussed when taking the history. The blood pressure is checked, preferably with the woman lying for a few minutes before. The spine should be checked for any tender areas as well as for longer term kyphosis and scoliosis, which might affect pelvic development, and the legs should be examined for oedema and varicose veins.

The abdomen is inspected for scars of previous operations—look carefully for laparoscopy scars below the umbilicus and for Pfannenstiel's incision above the pubis. Palpation is performed for masses other than the uterus—for example, fibroids and ovarian cysts. If the booking visit is before 12 weeks the uterus probably will not be felt on abdominal examination, but in a multiparous woman it may be; this should not cause the doctor to make any unnecessary comments about an enlarged uterus at this stage.

A vaginal assessment was traditionally performed at the booking visit. Its function was to confirm the soft enlargement of the uterus in pregnancy to try to assess the stage of gestation, to exclude other pelvic masses, to take a cervical smear, and to assess the bony pelvis. Many obstetricians now do not do a pelvic assessment at this stage; no woman likes having a vaginal examination and, if done in early pregnancy, it is associated in the woman's mind with any spontaneous miscarriage that may occur subsequently, even though it is irrelevant to the examination. A cervical smear test is incidental and opportunistic; it could be equally well done at the postnatal visit. Fetal size will be checked at 18-20 weeks by ultrasonography, but assessment of the bony pelvis is far better left until late pregnancy; firm palpation is required to perform this, and by 36 weeks the fetal presenting part is available for check against the inlet while the effect of progesterone on the pelvic ligaments is at its maximum. Furthermore, the woman by this time has more confidence in the antenatal staff and is more willing to have a vaginal examination.

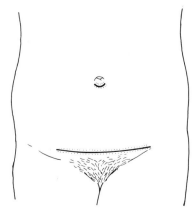

Laparoscopy and Pfannenstiel's scars.

Investigations

Venous blood is checked for:

● Haemoglobin concentration or mean cell volume (see chapter on Medical problems in pregnancy—II)

● ABO and rhesus groups and, if relevant, rhesus antibodies

● Antibodies to other blood groups—for example, Kell

● Haemoglobinopathies in women originating from Mediterranean, African, and West Indian countries

● α Fetoprotein concentrations for abnormality of the central nervous system or as part of a Down's syndrome screen (usually done at 16 weeks)

Normal antenatal management

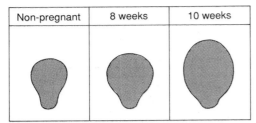

Non-pregnant	8 weeks	10 weeks

Growth of uterus in early pregnancy. Growth is usually in width rather than length, so the uterus seems fuller at first; it is also softer and has a cystic quality.

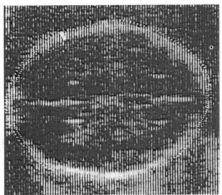

Ultrasound scan of fetal head showing the midline echo.

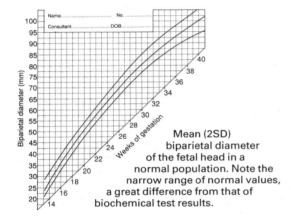

Mean (2SD) biparietal diameter of the fetal head in a normal population. Note the narrow range of normal values, a great difference from that of biochemical test results.

- Syphilis. A Wassermann reaction (WR) is non-specific; most clinics now use the *Treponema pallidum* haemagglutination test to investigate more specifically, but no test can be expected to differentiate syphilis from yaws or other treponematoses
- Rubella antibodies
- HIV antibodies. If the woman is at risk of infection through intravenous drug misuse, having received contaminated blood transfusions, or having a partner who is HIV positive she may request or be advised to have an HIV test. Full counselling should include her understanding the implications of both having the test and any positive result
- Hepatitis B antibodies
- Toxoplasmosis antibodies (if relevant)
- Cytomegalic virus antibodies (if relevant).

The urine is checked for:

- Protein
- Sugar
- Bacteria

Chest radiographs are rarely taken except in women from parts of the world where pulmonary tuberculosis is still endemic.

An ultrasound assessment is now performed on most women in the United Kingdom in pregnancy. It is best done at about 18-20 weeks to measure the biparietal diameter and so get a baseline value of fetal size and a confirmation of the stage of gestation to firm up the expected date of delivery.

At 18 weeks congenital abnormalities such as spina bifida, omphalocele, and abnormal kidneys may be excluded. A four chamber view of the heart is also possible at this stage to exclude gross abnormalities, but details of cardiac connections may not be obvious until 22-24 weeks. Other conditions which are characterised by decreased growth such as microcephaly or some forms of dwarfism may also not be apparent until late in the second trimester. Hence, though 16-18 weeks would be a useful time to assess gestational age by ultrasonography, much later assessments are needed to assess fetal normality. In addition, more highly skilled ultrasonographers and equipment of high resolution are needed to produce scans to enable assessment of normality. Many of these ultrasound studies of fetal anatomy have been developed in specialist units with highly skilled obstetric ultrasonographers. The ordinary ultrasound service at a district general hospital cannot be expected always to be able to provide such skill or equipment, although with increased training and better machines, some centres are now providing a fuller exclusion service at 20-24 weeks' gestation.

Subsequent antenatal visits

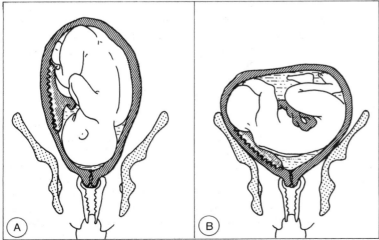

Lie of the fetus: (a) longitudinal lie, which is deliverable vaginally, and (b) transverse lie, which if it persists has to be delivered abdominally.

At each visit a short history is sought of events that have happened since the last antenatal clinic. The woman's weight is assessed, as is her blood pressure. These should be compared with the previous readings; proteinuria and glycosuria are excluded each time. Palpation of the abdomen and measurements of the fundus above the symphysis give a clinical guide to the rate of growth of the fetus, especially if they are performed at each visit by the same observer. In later weeks the lie and presentation of the fetus is assessed. In the last weeks of pregnancy the presenting part, which is usually the head, is checked against the pelvic inlet to ensure that it engages. If the fetal head is not engaged by 37 weeks it is helpful to see if it will engage. To do this, the head of the couch should be propped up to 60° from the horizontal and the lower abdomen re-examined. If this small change in entry angle

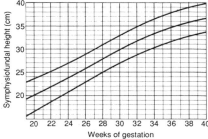

Mean (2SD) of symphysiofundal height by weeks of gestation. Note the wide range of readings for any given week of gestation and the even wider range of expected gestational weeks for any given reading.

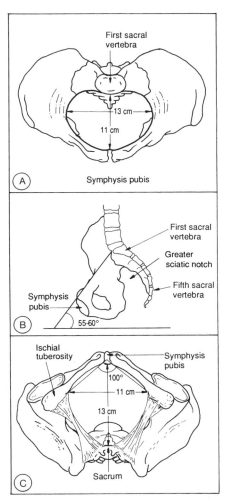

Outline of the bony pelvis. (a) Inlet seen from above, (b) side view showing angle of inclination, and (c) outlet seen from below.

Clinical assessment of bony pelvis should include checking the:

- Anteroposterior diameter from symphysis pubis to promontory of the sacrum (S1)
- Curve of the sacrum
- Prominence of the ischial spines
- Angle of the greater sciatic notch
- Width of the inferior border of the body of the pubis
- Subpubic angle

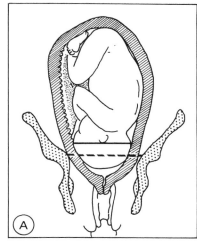
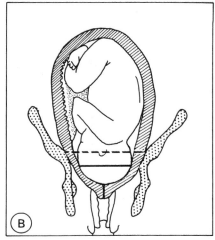

(a) The fetal head is not engaged as its maximum diameter (———) is above the inlet of the mother's pelvis (— — —). (b) The fetal head has descended so that its maximum diameter is below the inlet.

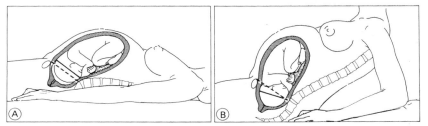

(a) The fetal head is not engaged, but when the mother sits up (b) gravity allows the head to sink below the inlet of the mother's pelvis so that the head will engage.

allows engagement of the fetal head it will usually go down with uterine contractions. This is a simple test giving useful information about the potential of the fetal head to negotiate the mother's pelvis; it deserves wider usage in antenatal clinics.

The amount of amniotic fluid is assessed clinically and if fetal movements are seen by the observer or reported by the mother, the fetal heart need not be auscultated at the antenatal clinic. If, however, the mother reports reduced movements the heart should be checked with a hand held Doppler fetal heart monitor or by cardiotocography so that the woman, too, can observe the regular beats and be reassured.

In a visit in the last few weeks of pregnancy a pelvic examination may be performed to check the bony pelvis, the points of importance being shown in the box. A well engaged fetal head after 36 weeks indicates, however, that the pelvis is adequate in this pregnancy and that any digital assessment is probably of theoretical value and need not be performed, but with a persistently non-engaged head or a breech presentation it should be done. Assessment of the cervix is wise at 32 weeks if the woman is at high risk of a preterm labour or is having a twin pregnancy; it is also useful to assess cervical ripeness if the pregnancy is postmature (after 42 weeks).

End of pregnancy

Traditionally in Britain many obstetricians have been concerned when a singleton pregnancy goes past 42 weeks. In the 1960s the actuarial risk of perinatal mortality did sharply increase after 41 weeks, but this is no longer so and the passage of 42 proved weeks is not used by all obstetricians as an indication for induction of labour. For example, if the cervix is not ripe it is unwise to induce merely on calendar dates. Instead, the unusually long length of gestation might be used as an indication for better and more frequent fetal surveillance rather than to take action, but this should be done at the consultant clinic in the hospital rather than in general practice.

Antenatal education

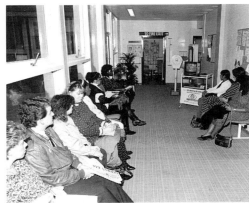

While waiting to see the doctor at the antenatal clinic women and their partners can learn about forthcoming events.

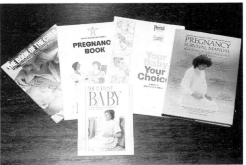

A wide variety of books on antenatal information is available.

Education and social benefits

The visits to an antenatal clinic can be a helpful time for the woman and her partner to learn about pregnancy. Formal antenatal education classes are held in most district hospitals, and couples are encouraged to attend a convenient course of instruction. Furthermore, informal discussions with midwives and doctors at the antenatal clinic are educational and much can be learnt from other mothers in the waiting time at the clinics. This is complemented by many excellent videos, which can be displayed in the antenatal waiting area.

Many good books exist about pregnancy and childbirth, offering a spectrum of styles and detail according to a woman's needs. A woman should be steered towards a well written account of what she needs in a form that best suits her lifestyle and religious observances and in a language that she can understand. Plenty of such books are now available, but all hospital and general practitioner obstetricians should read the material that is offered to the women who visit their clinics to make sure that they agree with and carry out what the books are saying.

In the welfare state of the United Kingdom pregnant women are entitled to several social security benefits, although in many ways this country lags behind many countries in the European Community. The doctor at the clinic would do well to read these from time to time as they change rapidly according to the whims of the Departments of Health and Social Security and of their political masters.

Conclusion

> Antenatal care is the cornerstone of obstetrics in this decade. Though the problems of labour are more dramatic and demand attention, many of them could be avoided by effective detection and management of antenatal variations from the normal

The antenatal visit in the community, general practice, surgery, or hospital should be friendly and held at a time when women can mix with others who are also pregnant and so informally discuss their problems. It also provides a nidus for antenatal education both formally at the antenatal classes and informally from staff and other women. The medical component is the core of the clinic and consists of the regular screening and assessment of symptomatic problems to bring the woman and her fetus to labour in the best state at the best time.

The tables of minimum care for multigravidas and additional visits for primigravidas are based on those in *Obstetrics* edited by A Turnbull and G Chamberlain and published by Churchill Livingstone. The distribution of length of gestation is reproduced by permission of Butterworth Heinemann from *British Births 1970* by R Chamberlain and G Chamberlain.

CHECKING FOR FETAL WELLBEING

Perinatal mortality in England and Wales in 1983 according to various maternal factors

Maternal factor	Rate per 1000 total births
Age:	
<16	26·9
16-20	13·4
21-24	10·1
25-30	9·5
31-35	9·8
>35	13·8
Parity:	
0	11·0
1	7·0
2	8·0
3	8·5
≥4	16·0
Socioeconomic class:	
I	7·3
II	8·5
IIIN	9·0
IIIM	9·9
IV	12·5
V	12·7
Place of birth:	
United Kingdom	10·2
Republic of Ireland	7·9
India	13·3
Africa	12·0
West Indies	11·2
Pakistan	20·2

The great reduction in maternal mortality and morbidity in the past 20 years allows more attention to be concentrated on the fetus during antenatal care. Perinatal mortality has been reduced, but still in England and Wales out of 100 babies born, one will die around the time of birth, two have an abnormality, and six have a birth weight under 2500 g. With smaller family sizes in the Western world, parents expect a perfect result. General practitioners and obstetricians are performing more thorough checks to try to detect the fetuses that are likely to be at increased risk. These investigations do not replace clinical examination but provide the fine tuning of assessment. The mother still needs, however, to see someone who can talk to her and discuss the implications and results of these new tests with her.

Some groups of women are at high risk because of their medicosocial background. The extremes of maternal age (under 20 and over 35), high parity (over four pregnancies), low socioeconomic class (Office of Population Censuses and Surveys classes IV and V), and some racial groups (Pakistan born women) seem to confer a higher actuarial risk on the babies born to such women. Consequently these women deserve extra antenatal surveillance to detect a fetus with variations from normal. Others show poor growth of the fetus in the latter days of pregnancy or develop raised blood pressure during pregnancy, two manifestations of a poor flow to the placental bed. Such fetuses have a poor nutritional reserve—a decreased blood flow to the placental bed reduces the amounts of nutrients in pregnancy and of oxygen in labour. A series of tests have been developed; some of these are screening tests best applied to the total antenatal population or to a subset considered to be at higher risk. Other tests are diagnostic and specifically used for women with babies thought to be compromised clinically.

Tests in early pregnancy (up to 13 weeks)

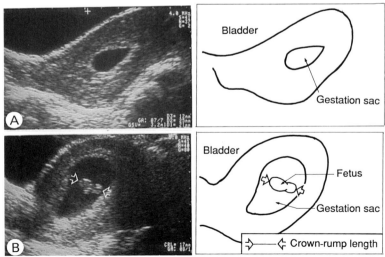

(a) The embryonic sac can be seen at six weeks of gestation in decidua. As yet no fetal parts can be identified.

(b) The same sac two weeks later. Fetal parts can easily be seen between the arrows. The pulsation of the fetal heart may also be seen at this time.

Ultrasonography—The earliest in pregnancy that the embryo may be visualised by abdominal ultrasonography is six to seven weeks; it may be shown a little earlier with a vaginal probe. At six weeks the embryonic sac can be seen but embryonic tissue cannot be confidently visualised, even with machines of high resolution and skilled ultrasonographers. By seven to eight weeks most ultrasound machines should be able to show the embryo and a fetal heart pulse can often be seen.

Checking for fetal wellbeing

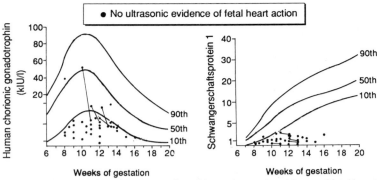

Hormone concentrations in pregnancies with no ultrasonic evidence of fetal heart action. Left: Serum concentrations of human chorionic gonadotrophin. Values usually rise sharply to reach a maximum at about 10-12 weeks and decline after this. They seem to relate to fetal wellbeing and are used as a measure of fetal state in the first few weeks of pregnancy. Right: Maternal serum concentrations of Schwangerschaftsprotein 1. This protein is made by the fetus and placenta and concentrations increase steadily through pregnancy. Many fetuses who abort have concentrations below the 10th centile in the first weeks of gestation.

Hormone tests are currently being developed that may be helpful in very early pregnancy to detect women who are likely to miscarry early. They mostly measure proteins derived from the placenta—for example, human chorionic gonadotrophin and Schwangerschaftsprotein 1. Several other proteins are measurable, but these two have been most researched. Oestrogen and progesterone tests are too non-specific to be of prognostic value so early in gestation.

Chorionic villus sampling is at present mainly used to detect chromosomal abnormalities and is considered in the next chapter.

Tests in mid-pregnancy (14-28 weeks)

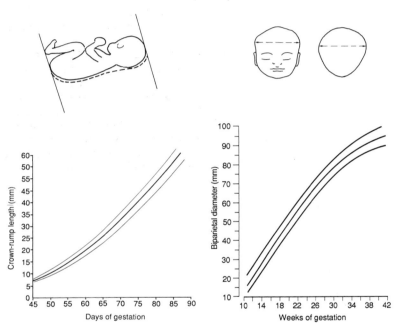

Crown-rump length by days of gestation and biparietal diameter by weeks of gestation show a narrow range inside 2SD of the mean, indicating a good test.

Ultrasonography has become a more sophisticated tool in the past 15 years, so that by 20 weeks of pregnancy the fetus can be visualised precisely. Two distinct sets of measurements are taken of the fetus to assess growth and detect malformations. The detection of malformations is the subject of the next chapter.

Growth may be determined by assessment of a series of measurements of the individual fetus at different times in pregnancy. These may then be compared with a background population to see whether the fetus is growing at the same rate as a statistically comparable group of its peers. Obviously the growth chart should relate to a population from which the fetus comes and not be taken from another population mix, although growth charts generated by ultrasonography are similar for many races except Asians.

Crown-rump length—From seven to 12 weeks the length of the embryo's body can be measured precisely from the crown of the head to the tip of the rump. This measurement is helpful in dating the maturity of an embryo or early fetus, but after 12 weeks it becomes less reliable because the fetus flexes and extends to a greater degree.

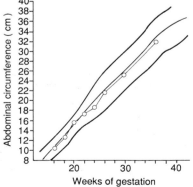

Abdominal circumference by weeks of gestation showing the mean (2SD). The variation is slightly wider than that in biparietal diameter but growth rates are almost linear until 40 weeks.

Biparietal diameter—The distance between the two parietal eminences of the skull gives a precise measurement of fetal head size. From about 16 weeks the range of variation in a normal population widens so that in the last trimester this measurement is less useful. Early biparietal measurements are extremely helpful in dating the pregnancy with more precision even than using the date of the last menstrual period when the woman is certain of her dates. Currently, this is probably the most commonly used technique of ultrasound fetal monitoring in the Western world.

Abdominal circumference—Measurement of the fetal waist at the level of the umbilical vein provides a good assessment of the size of the fetal liver. Poor fetal nutrition prevents adequate growth of the liver following the failure to lay down glycogen. Serial measurements of abdominal circumference (or area) give good warning of placental insufficiency. A fetus who is growing well is unlikely to die except from an acute event.

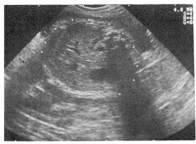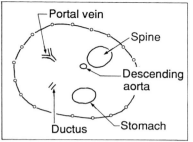

Late in pregnancy fetal growth can be detected by examining the fetal abdomen, and the circumference can be marked out (by a series of dots).

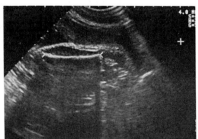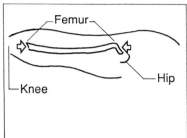

Femur length (between two arrow heads) can be measured easily by ultrasonography.

Femur length can be readily measured from about 12 until 40 weeks. It allows a check on the somatic growth of the fetus. Impaired femur growth occurs with skeletal dysplasia.

Amniotic fluid volume—The estimation of amniotic fluid volume is a measure of fetal metabolism. Volume is assessed by measuring the height of the largest vertical column of fluid detected by ultrasonography. A column less than 2 cm near term indicates poor production of amniotic fluid (oligohydramnios).

All these five measurements have different uses at different times of pregnancy.

Measurements of the biparietal diameter and femur should be used for assessing gestational age. Growth is best assessed by serial circumference measurements of the fetal head and abdomen. In late pregnancy fetal weight is estimated by using all variables. Assessment of amniotic fluid is an attempt to study dynamic changes as it reflects fetal urine production; this is decreased in placental underperfusion.

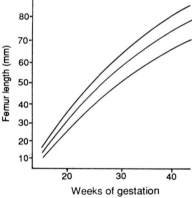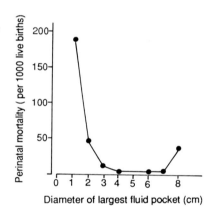

Growth in femur length by weeks of pregnancy showing mean (2SD).

The relation of amniotic fluid volume to perinatal mortality. Low fluid volumes (vertical diameter of largest pocket <2 cm) are associated with a high mortality.

Tests in late pregnancy (29-40 weeks)

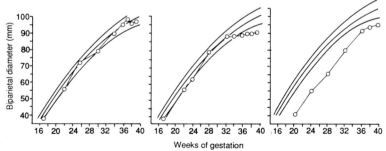

Biparietal diameter during pregnancy. Left: Growth follows the normal range of variation and stays within 2SD of the mean. Middle: Growth tails off from about 32 weeks, the head growing hardly at all in the last weeks. Right: The first reading at 20 weeks is well outside the normal range. If the readings are put back four weeks growth falls inside the normal range. The woman in this case was probably incorrect in her dates.

One of the main signs of fetal wellbeing in late pregnancy is continued growth, measured by serial ultrasound examination of abdominal area, femur length, or biparietal diameter. Readings from early pregnancy are needed to give a baseline to the growth measurements in the third trimester. This method of monitoring fetal growth has a high predictive power—that is, high sensitivity and specificity.

Checking for fetal wellbeing

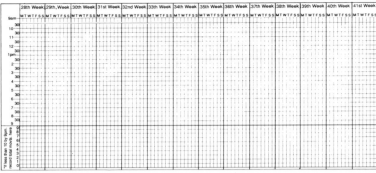

Cardiff "count to ten" kick chart. The timing of fetal movements can be graphically displayed on this chart by the mother, who is asked to contact the hospital if there are <10 movements in 12 hours.

Movements

The movements of the fetus are detected by the mother from about 20 weeks. In the last 10 weeks of pregnancy they may be used as a coarse measure of fetal wellbeing. Many women feel individual movements distinctly; they record these on a "count to ten" kick chart, which estimates how long it takes for the fetus to make 10 movements. In most cases this happens within the first hour or two of the observation period, but fewer than 10 movements in 12 hours may be an early warning sign of problems. The woman should report to her obstetric department for more intensive testing, usually cardiotocography.

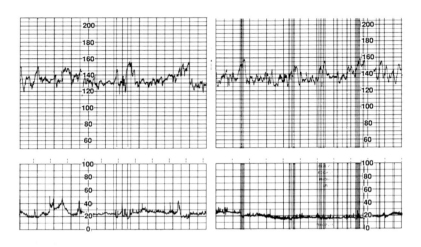

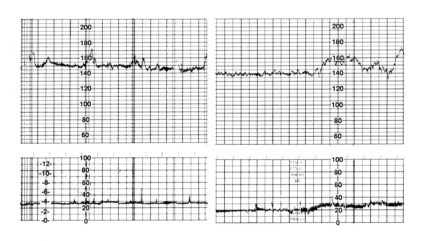

Cardiotocography

The fetal heart rate bears some relation to the body's response to lack of oxygen—hypoxaemia. This may be measured from 28 weeks by an external ultrasound transmitter and receiver attached to a recording system. The changes in the fetal heart rate in relation to events external to the heart rate such as uterine contractions or fetal movements can be assessed.

The baseline is important, a bradycardia being a warning sign. Episodic changes are more commonly seen, the most hopeful being an acceleration; decelerations are of serious import.

Heart rate varies with the balance of the sympathetic and parasympathetic nervous systems, the activity of chemoreceptors in the aorta, and concentrations of adrenaline and acetylcholine. In consequence, when the fetus is awake baseline variability is normal. Reduced variability so that the trace becomes flat is a sign that the heart is not responding to the interaction of stimuli. This may mean accumulation of metabolic catabolites—that is, fetal acidosis. Sleep patterns need to be excluded from this diagnosis, particularly in less mature babies, as a flat trace can occur for 40 minutes or so when the fetus is asleep. The easiest way to distinguish the two is to wake the baby up by asking the mother to move around and repeat the test an hour later.

Other sinister changes include episodic decelerations with uterine contractions and a solitary long deceleration lasting for over five minutes.

Cardiotocograph records are widely used in the United Kingdom to monitor women at high risk in the last days of pregnancy to determine the best time for delivering the baby. Because of the poor prognostic value of the individual variables that make up an antenatal cardiotocograph trace, their precise value in prediction is hard to define. A severely abnormal trace probably indicates action but an apparently normal one should not blinker decisions. The trace should be considered with other data from the pregnancy and rarely be regarded as a solitary indicant for induction.

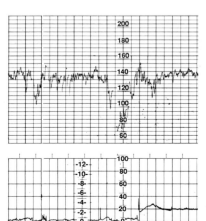

Antenatal cardiotocography showing fetal heart rate above and uterine pressure below in each trace. Top left: Normal fetal heart rate with a lot of baseline variability. Top right: Fetal movements (shown by the vertical bars) are accompanied by accelerations in the heart rate. Middle left: The heart rate shows low variability, implying that the fetus is asleep. Middle right: The fetus is asleep but wakes at the end of the trace. Left: The heart rate shows episodic decelerations, which have a bad prognosis.

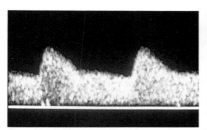
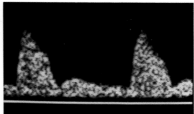

Doppler studies showing the waveforms of normal (left) and narrowed (right) arcuate arteries of the placental bed.

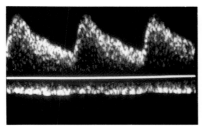
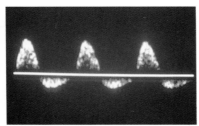

Left: Normal waveforms of the umbilical artery. Right: Severely abnormal waveforms of the umbilical artery showing reduced and even reversed flow in the diastolic phase, which suggests that the fetus is compromised.

Doppler studies

The flow of blood in the arcuate branches of the uterine artery on the maternal side of the placental bed and in the umbilical artery on the fetal side can be measured by the Doppler principle. Ultrasound waves are beamed in and their reflected echo patterns vary with flow. This method of monitoring is still mostly at the research stage, but the interpretation of patterns is beginning to show that it is useful clinically. Abnormal waveforms from the arcuate artery are useful in predicting which women will develop severe hypertension in pregnancy. In a fetus shown to be small by ultrasound measurements the umbilical artery waveforms help to identify the truly pathological from the constitutionally small baby. Absence of or reversal of flow in the umbilical artery during diastole carries a 25-40% mortality, and up to a quarter of survivors have substantial morbidity. Conversely, small fetuses with normal umbilical waveforms have a good outcome. Regional blood flow in fetal carotid and renal arteries is being researched as it too may reflect fetal wellbeing.

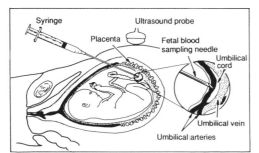

Cordocentesis.

Invasive studies

In the second half of pregnancy fetal blood may be sampled by cordocentesis, when the oxygen saturation, carbon dioxide concentration, and concentrations of non-volatile bases such as lactate and pyruvate are measured in small blood samples. Blood is removed from the umbilical vein in the cord close to the fetus; the procedure carries a 1-2% risk of fetal death but the results can be invaluable about the state of fetal acid-base and oxygen concentrations. Furthermore, in some cases chromosome studies on the leucocytes yield important results.

Fetuses used to be examined structurally in late pregnancy by fetoscopy, but ultrasonography has now mostly replaced it. Fetoscopy is still helpful, however, in detecting problems of the face and limbs, which can be visualised readily in women at high risk of such problems. If a woman has previously given birth to a child with a hare lip and cleft palate she will be greatly relieved to know that any subsequent children are not affected. It is thus helpful treatment for a small number of mothers.

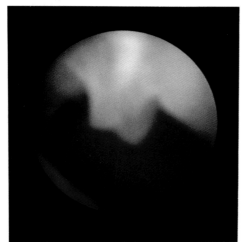

View through a fetoscope of the back of a fetal hard palate and uvula. Though the uvula is slightly bifid, there is no cleft. This photograph reassured the mother, who was terrified of having another child with a harelip and cleft palate.

Hormone concentrations

In late pregnancy the hormone tests for fetal wellbeing have mostly been put to one side. The estimation of oestriol concentration (or total oestrogens) in the mother's urine or blood in late pregnancy was used to give some idea of the state of the fetoplacental unit. Unfortunately, the wide variance of results inside the normal range did not allow precise enough prediction and the tests have mostly been replaced by biophysical ones. In a woman at high risk, however, a series of oestrogen estimations considered longitudinally may guide the obstetrician who still believes in these tests.

Testing for progesterone and human placental lactogen has mostly suffered the same fate as that for oestrogen, for the same reasons.

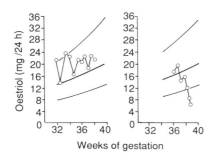

Urinary oestriol concentrations (mean (2SD)) during gestation. The range is much greater than that of biophysical tests. Left: Variation during a normal pregnancy. Right: Acute placental malfunction in a woman with hypertension. Currently, signs of fetal compromise measured biophysically would have indicated that she be delivered before the last oestriol readings were available.

Conclusions

> Fetal investigations should be considered to be either screening, for use in large populations, or specifically diagnostic, for use in a selected number of fetuses in which there is clinical suspicion of significant pathological lesions

The clinical assessment of the fetus can be extended by a series of tests. Some are simple and easy to do and are used as screening tests on the whole antenatal population—for example, ultrasonography for checking fetal growth. Most fetal investigations, however, should be kept for women who are at high risk of specific conditions—for example, amniocentesis for women at risk of Down's syndrome.

The development of more complex biophysical tests has led to a concentration of antenatal care for women at high risk in certain hospital units, as even many district general hospitals do not have all the facilities required. In consequence, proper use of regional centres for specialist tests must be encouraged. It may be unpleasant for the woman to have to move from her home area to a centre 40 or 60 km away, but this is usually acceptable if benefits of fetal diagnosis and treatment can be explained by the family practitioner so that the woman realises she is helping her baby. Unfortunately, resources and skills cannot be spread uniformly throughout the country. A natural resistance to the new happens in medicine, but it is Luddite to ignore new investigations merely because they were developed after the practitioner qualified.

The figure showing concentrations of human chorionic gonadotrophin and Schwangerschaftsprotein 1 is reproduced by permission of Blackwell Scientific Publications from Westergaard JG, Teisner B, Sinosich MJ, Madsen LT, Grudzinskas JG, *British Journal of Obstetrics and Gynaecology* 1985;**92**:77-83. The figure showing the relation between amniotic fluid volume and perinatal mortality is reproduced by permission of the W B Saunders Company from *Maternal Fetal Medicine* edited by R Creasy and R Resnick.

I thank Mr Malcolm Pearce for the photographs of Doppler waveforms, and Professor Charles Rodeck for the photograph taken through a fetoscope.

Recommended reading
Chamberlain G, ed. *Modern antenatal care of the fetus.* Oxford: Blackwell Scientific Publications, 1990.

DETECTION AND MANAGEMENT OF CONGENITAL ABNORMALITIES

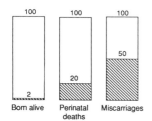

Proportions of congenital abnormalities in various populations.

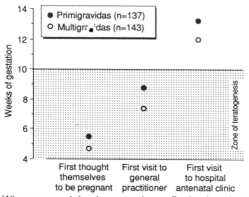

When women joined antenatal care. By the time they arrived in the hospital clinic it was far too late for advice to have any influence on the embryo in the first trimester.

A congenital abnormality in their forthcoming baby is greatly feared by couples; we are not many generations away from the superstitious who looked on malformation as a retribution for misbehaviour. Congenital abnormalities are one of the major causes of perinatal mortality and morbidity.

The known causes of abnormality are genetic or environmental. Genetic abnormality depends on the chromosomes we get from our parents together with the breaks and realignments occurring at fertilisation. Maternal aging increases the risk of abnormalities in genes. A good account of genetic abnormalities is found in the recent *ABC of Clinical Genetics*.

Environmental factors interfere wth embryonic development at a precise stage of organogenesis. They are difficult to pinpoint and often are misassociated. Obvious insults such as exposure to thalidomide, *x* rays, and rubella can be identified; more difficult is the precise place of factors such as organic solvents in the cleaning industry and viral infections such as chickenpox.

An antenatal service should aim at diagnosing congenital abnormalities as early as possible. Though the ideal treatment is prevention, this is usually too late by the time the woman joins the antenatal clinic. If an abnormality can be detected early the couple may be offered the choice of a termination of pregnancy. This is allowed under statutory grounds E of the modified Abortion Act 1967, and 1619 abortions occurred in England and Wales in 1990 for this reason.

Not all couples want to abort their unborn child even if it has an abnormality. Antenatal diagnostic facilities should be made available not only to those who agree to a termination of pregnancy if an abnormality is found but to all affected couples for the following reasons:-

● It gives the couple more time to accustom themselves and other children in the family to the idea that an abnormal child is to be born

● If the abnormality is not lethal, early diagnosis allows plans to be made for the woman to be delivered in a centre where full treatment may be given early

● Certain abnormalities that entail back pressure on essential organs such as the kidneys may be amenable to intrauterine decompression operations. This is less useful than first thought for, although the immediate physical pressure can be relieved, there are often underlying abnormalities of the organs themselves which lead to poor results in the long term.

In the early 1990s antenatal screening for congenital abnormalities is mostly concerned with the detection of malformations of the central nervous system and abnormalities of chromosomal origin. In special groups other fetal conditions such as cystic fibrosis and limb malformations are sought.

Modified certificate A of the Abortion Act 1967. Revised 1991.

Testing in early pregnancy

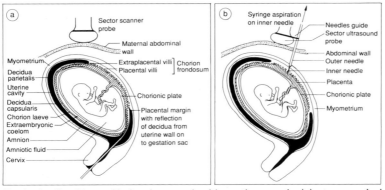

Chorionic villus biopsy. Under ultrasound guidance there can be (*a*) a transcervical approach of the cannula to the edge of the developing placenta or (*b*) a transabdominal aspiration by needle from the middle of the trophoblast mass.

Chromosomal problems

To examine fetal chromosomes a few cells are required. In chorionic villus sampling a minute piece of trophoblast tissue is removed for examination of the chromosomes in the cell nucleus and, with increasing confidence, DNA assessment. Such sampling is commonly performed at 9-11 weeks of gestation, and a preliminary result is available a couple of days after the test and confirmed about three weeks later (compared with the delay of at least 21 days for amniocentesis). Sampling is under ultrasound control by the transcervical or the transabdominal route, depending on the site of placental implantation. Recent reports of fetal damage being associated with the transabdominal approach have led to a reduction in its use.[1]

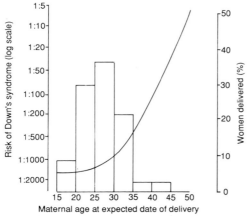

Risks of Down's syndrome. The risk increases after 35 and sharply after 40. The percentage of women in the United Kingdom who deliver by each age group is also shown. Although the risk is high after 40, the numbers of women delivering are small.

The apparent attraction of early chorionic villus sampling and its quicker result are offset by the higher risks of stimulating a miscarriage. Abortion rates associated with chorionic villus sampling are 2-4% compared with 0·3-1·0% with amniocentesis. At 10 weeks of gestation, however, the rate of spontaneous miscarriage is biologically much higher than at 16 weeks, so the comparison is not only of techniques. Many obstetrics units are now using chorionic villus sampling for women at high risk, and with experience the miscarriage rates would be expected to fall.

A nationally organised randomised controlled trial is in process to sort out the comparative advantages of chorionic villus sampling and amniocentesis. Generally it found that chorionic villus sampling had more problems than amniocentesis in diagnostic accuracy, safety, and the need for further testing.[2] However, the obvious advantages of earlier testing and receiving a quicker answer must be weighed against this. Doctors would do well to refer women asking for either procedure to a department of obstetrics that performs both and will give impartial and balanced advice in each individual case.

Trisomy 21 (Down's syndrome) is much commoner in women over 35, but still half of the babies with this condition are born to women under that age. Although the risks to mothers under 35 are less, the number of babies is much greater. To negate this, simple screening is required as both chorionic villus sampling and amniocentesis are unsuitable and invasive procedures that are very labour intensive. Hence the recent work assessing a combination of biochemical tests of maternal blood in early pregnancy to screen for Down's syndrome is of wide interest. Maternal α fetoprotein, human chorionic gonadotrophin, and oestriol concentrations are measured and compared with background data derived from large populations. The predictive value of the combination of tests is high about three times greater than using age alone; this allows a population that is at high risk of Down's syndrome to be pinpointed. If that risk is greater than one in 100, it is then recommended that amniocentesis be performed to assess the fetal chromosomes. This test is new but is being tried in some health districts and has great promise of screening for Down's syndrome in younger mothers. However, it is not a diagnostic test—as is sighting a trisomy of chromosome 21—and provides only a measure of risk.

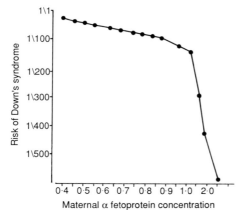

The risk of Down's syndrome in a woman of 40 according to serum α fetoprotein concentration at 14-20 weeks. The actuarial risk by age in a woman of 40 is 1:100.

Testing in mid-pregnancy

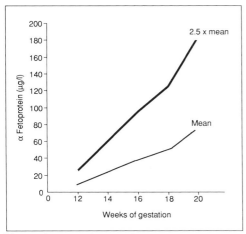

Maternal serum α fetoprotein concentration by weeks of gestation. The upper line is taken as the boundary of the normal group so it is important to date the pregnancy precisely—that is, by ultrasound measurement of the biparietal diameter.

Structural abnormalities

Open neural tube defects such as anencephaly and open spina bifida allow α fetoprotein to escape from cerebral spinal fluid into the amniotic fluid, whence it is absorbed into the maternal blood, producing higher than normal concentrations. This is the basis of α fetoprotein screening performed between 14 and 16 weeks. It is virtually non-invasive, entailing only taking a blood sample, and has a high predictive value. Fetal gestational age must be estimated by ultrasonography. False positive results can be caused by multiple pregnancy, a dead fetus, bleeding behind the placenta (which may manifest as a threatened abortion), and a few rather rarer abnormalities of the fetus such as gastroschisis.

If the serum α fetoprotein concentration is high either an amniotic fluid sample can be obtained by amniocentesis to measure α fetoprotein concentration or acetylcholinesterase activity, which is more specific, or a special ultrasound scan is performed to examine the spine and head carefully at 18-19 weeks of gestation.

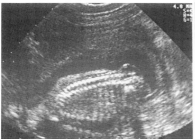
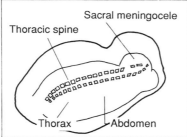

Ultrasound scan of a fetus with a sacral meningocele taken at 19 weeks.

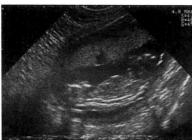
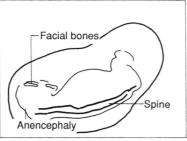

Scan of a fetus with anencephaly taken at 17 weeks.

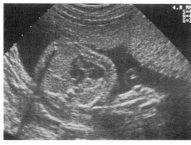
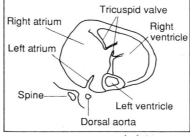

Ultrasound scan of the heart of a fetus with mitral atresia taken at 23 weeks' gestation.

By 20 weeks the fetus can be seen clearly on ultrasonography and many neural tube defects will have been detected. A little later the heart can be examined and the four chambers identified so that major cardiac abnormalities can be excluded. Limbs can be seen to exclude any shortening and, if relevant, the sex of the child may be determined by sighting the external genitalia in the male.

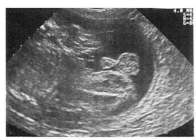
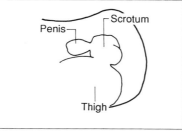

Ultrasound scan showing male genitalia resting on the section of the thigh in a fetus of 30 weeks.

Congenital abnormalities

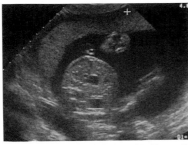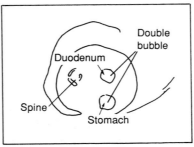

Double bubble effect of duodenal atresia, with the lower bubble in the stomach and the upper bubble in the duodenum. Normally continuity can be traced between these two bubbles.

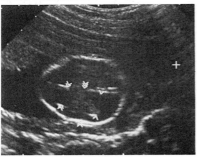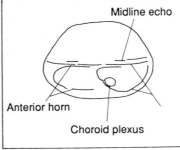

Hydrocephalus showing enlarged posterior horn of the ventricle (between single arrows) and anterior horn (between double arrows).

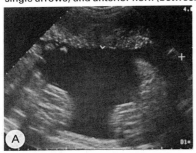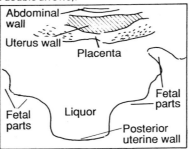

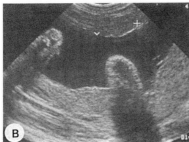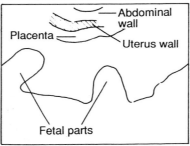

Amniotic fluid estimation. (a) The largest pool has the longest column of 5·3 cm (between the arrows). (b) In polyhydramnios the longest pool between the arrows has a column of 9·1 cm. Generally 8·0 cm is taken as the upper limit of normal.

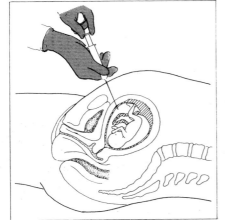

Amniocentesis under local anaesthesia. The fluid withdrawn (about 10 ml) is spun down and either the cells are used for culture or the supernatant is used to estimate concentrations of α fetoprotein.

Later still the kidneys may be assessed for cysts or damming back of urine, producing hydronephrosis. Blockage in the intestinal tract can be checked by the presence of bubbles of fluid in the stomach, duodenal, or large bowel area. The cerebral cortex and ventricles can also be easily visualised and measured.

The volume of amniotic fluid can be calculated from measurements inside the uterine cavity or more pragmatically by measuring the longest column at the maximum diameter of the largest fluid pool. The placenta can be seen and its function assessed from the degree of degenerative changes occurring in the last weeks of pregnancy, but this is a non-specific test.

These investigations permit a thorough knowledge of the unborn child. Most of the skills are available in the ultrasound departments of district general hospitals, but there is more expert back up at the special obstetric ultrasound clinics of regional teaching hospitals.

Chromosomal abnormalities

In mid-pregnancy the chromosomal state of the fetus may be checked from cells removed at amniocentesis. It is difficult but not impossible to get enough fetal cells before 16 weeks, but with new techniques of DNA amplification fewer cells will suffice so amniocentesis could be possible two or three weeks earlier. It takes three weeks to culture cells in the laboratory and so no chromosomal results can be given after amniocentesis for at least 21 days.

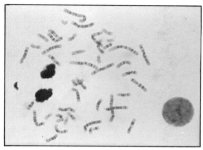 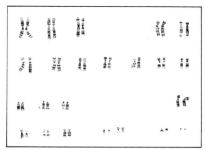

Metaphase spread of chromosome material from a nucleus after culture. The chromosomes are photographed and the print cut out and arranged in pairs to show the normal arrangement for a female, two X chromosomes at the end of the bottom grouping.

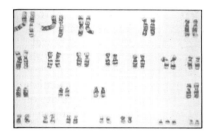

Chromosomes of a woman with trisomy 21. The last but one grouping (position 21) has three chromosomes instead of two.

The commonest use of amniocentesis is for the diagnosis of Down's syndrome (trisomy 21), and in most parts of England and Wales women over the age of 35 are offered this screening test. Perhaps in future screening of plasma concentrations of hormones and steroids may be used as an indicator for a chromosomal check. Amniocentesis is an invasive procedure with a small risk of spontaneous abortion (0·3-1·0% above background rate of miscarriage within a few days). This risk is very much less if the procedure is done under ultrasound guidance by an experienced obstetrician (0·3-0·5%). There is a very small risk of infection, which is avoided by proper antiseptic techniques.

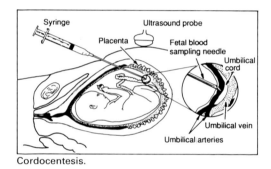

Cordocentesis.

Occasionally from about 20 weeks of pregnancy it is necessary to be certain that the fetus has normal chromosomes if a high risk pregnancy is to be continued under adverse circumstances. It is wise to know that the baby is normal before putting the mother through many weeks of often unpleasant treatment and possibly a caesarean section. The white cells of fetal blood can be obtained at cordocentesis by penetrating the umbilical cord where the vessels are held firmest, close to the placenta. Chromosome examination of the white blood cells gives a result fairly speedily (two to four days).

Availability of tests

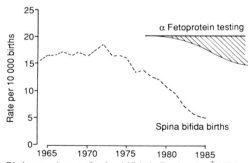

Birth prevalence of spina bifida in England and Wales. A slight reduction has occurred from the mid-1960s, becoming sharper from 1973. Testing for α fetoprotein, although described in the early 1970s, was not widespread in its use until the late 1970s and so there may be a coincident factor in this reduction as well as the effect of screening. Many would think this is due to an improved diet for the women of the country.

Biochemical screening for abnormalities of the central nervous system and for Down's syndrome is patchy and varies from one district health authority to another. The reasons lie not just in the whims of economic dictate but with variations in the interpretation of epidemiological data.

Abnormalities of the central nervous system

The total number of abnormalities of the central nervous system in England and Wales has fallen since the early 1970s. Data are based on three sources:

- Notification of termination of pregnancy for abnormalities of the central nervous system
- Death certification of stillbirths and neonatal deaths because of abnormalities
- Notifications of abnormalities of babies who live.

There is a differential in the south of Britain, where the proportional decrease is even greater. In many parts of England, particularly in the four metropolitan regional health authorities, the rate of abnormalities of the central nervous system is less than one per 1000. At this level a screening programme that used α fetoprotein might do more harm than good because action might be taken on false positive results. Many authorities have abandoned screening for these reasons. Ultrasonography as a screening test for anencephaly has good results, and when modern, high resolution equipment is available spina bifida can be detected. Although the special skills and equipment are currently not always available in ultrasonography clinics, the state of affairs should improve.

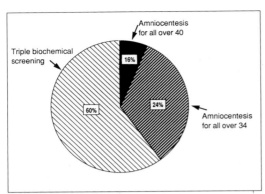

Detection rates of Down's syndrome comparing age as the only criterion with the results of triple biochemistry screening to indicate amniocentesis.

Down's syndrome

As explained previously, the risks of Down's syndrome are greater in women over 35, but because most babies are born to women under this age about half of the babies with the syndrome will be missed if age is used as an indicator for fetal chromosome tests. The use of triple biochemical screening with ultrasonography may answer this, although costs will have to be considered. In one health district in south London it costs £38 000 a year to diagnose Down's syndrome in one fetus. Some health authorities would set this against the cost of maintaining a child born with Down's syndrome for the rest of his or her life in an institution, probably over £500 000. The cost of diagnosis, however, comes from one year's budget, whereas the cost of maintenance is spread over many years' budgets in the future; local health authorities are forced into this philosophical financial juggling.

If triple biochemistry screening with ultrasonography is introduced some women considered to be at high risk by age alone will be reallotted to a lower risk group on the results of the triple biochemistry screening. Thus eventually the number of amniocenteses and chromosome examinations will be reduced, but there will be difficulty in persuading such conservative groups of people as patients and doctors to abandon the age indication for the newer biochemical screening of risk. This subject is full of promise, and new indices may add even further precision to the screening—for example, femur length, which is commonly shorter in fetuses with trisomy 21.

Conclusions

> Detection of fetal abnormalities in early pregnancy need not just lead to termination of pregnancy. Many results confirm normality and so reassure the mother. Even when positive, the results lead to the provision of better neonatal services when the affected baby is born

At first the antenatal detection of congenital abnormalities may seem to lead only to a nihilistic outcome, but the diagnosis can lead to other lines of management such as the preparation for early paediatric surgery or, in future, to genetic engineering. This is unlikely to be of any help once the embryo has started its development, but work done now on formed embryos can be extrapolated back to research on the oocyte. Here recombinant DNA technology may be used to change the affected part of a chromosome before cell development starts, thus producing a normal fetus. Such technology obviously needs to be controlled by society to help couples who previously had no chance of producing a normal baby.

I thank Dr Rashmi Patel for providing the ultrasound material shown in this chapter, and Dr J Taylor of the karyometric laboratory at St George's Hospital for the chromosome illustrations. The data for birth prevalence of spina bifida in England and Wales are reproduced by permission of Churchill Livingstone from *Obstetrics* edited by A Turnbull and G Chamberlain.

1 Firth HV, Boyd TA, Chamberlain P, Mackenzie IZ, Linderbaun RH, Huson SM. Severe limb abnormalities after chorion villus sampling at 56-66 days' gestation. *Lancet* 1991;**337**:762-3.
2 MRC Working Party on the Evaluation of Chorion Villus Sampling. Medical Research Council European trial of chorion villus sampling. *Lancet* 1991;**337**:1492-9.

Recommended reading
Whittle M, Connor MJ. *Prenatal diagnosis.* Oxford: Blackwell Scientific Publications, 1989.

WORK IN PREGNANCY

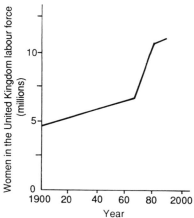

Numbers of women in the labour force in the United Kingdom.

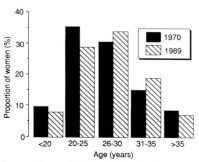

Proportions of births in England and Wales by maternal age in 1970 and 1989.

Both the proportions and numbers of women in the paid workforce have been increasing in England and Wales since before the second world war. By the year 2000 half of the workforce will be women; many may be in part time posts but this statistic has important implications for childbearing and reproduction.

Other important changes are women working longer in pregnancy and the postponement of starting a family to an older age. Most couples need two incomes to pay the mortgage and other loans. When the woman becomes pregnant she receives maternity benefits, but these are poor compared with those in other European countries and income will be reduced.

In the United Kingdom the number of women over the age of 25 having babies has increased in the past 20 years because the years of reproduction are those of career advancement and each pregnancy becomes a gap in climbing the ladder of promotion.

About half of the women in the paid workforce currently continue to work longer into pregnancy than women did in the 1960s. Whereas some stop around the 28th week of pregnancy, three quarters of them continue into the 34th or 35th week. Women are entitled to maternity leave for six weeks on full pay and 12 weeks on half. This can start from 11 weeks before the expected time of delivery, as certified by a doctor or midwife on the MATB1 form. Most women, however, prefer to have as much time as possible with their newborn child after delivery and so do not leave work early.

In certain circumstances a woman leaving her job during pregnancy is entitled to return after maternity leave up to one year after delivery. The employer must, however, employ more than five people and the woman must have worked with the employer for two years in a full time job or longer in a part time post. If she wishes to protect her job she must give her employer 21 days' notice of her intent to stop working and she cannot leave until the 28th week of pregnancy. In return for this the employer must keep the job open for a year and, though the exact job may not be there, a job of an equivalent nature must be offered.

Average maternity payments in Europe

Country	Allowance/ week (£)	Duration (weeks)
Belgium	137	14
Denmark	131	28
France	150	16
West Germany	179	14
Greece	90	14
Republic of Ireland	125	14
Italy	143	44
Luxembourg	179	16
The Netherlands	179	12
Portugal	179	14
Spain	134	14
United Kingdom	31	18

MATERNITY CERTIFICATE MAT B1

Please fill in this form in ink
Name of patient

TO THE PATIENT
Please read the notes on the back of this form ▶

Fill in this part if you are giving the certificate before the confinement.
Do not fill this in more than 14 weeks before the week when the baby is expected.
I certify that I examined you on the date given below. In my opinion you can expect to have your baby in the week that includes ...... /........ /......
We use week to mean the 7 days starting on a Sunday and ending on a Saturday.

Fill in this part if you are giving the certificate after the confinement.
I certify that I attended you in connection with the birth which took place on ...... /........ /...... when you were delivered of a child [ ] children
In my opinion your baby was expected in the week that includes ...... /........ /......

Date of examination ...... /........ /......
Date of signing ...... /........ /......
Signature

Registered midwives
Please give your UKCC PIN here

Doctors
Please stamp your name and address here if the form has not been stamped by the Family Practitioner Committee.

MATB1 form.

Work in pregnancy
Types of work

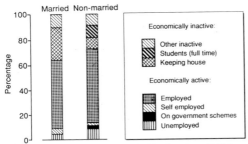

Working status of women in England and Wales in 1986.

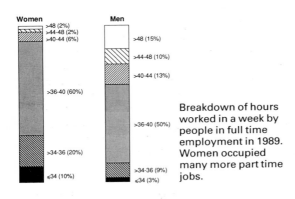

Breakdown of hours worked in a week by people in full time employment in 1989. Women occupied many more part time jobs.

It is an implicit and undiscussed assumption (by men) that any woman who works outside the home will continue to keep house as well. Hence housework must be considered first when examining work in pregnancy. All women work in the house, where there is washing, cooking, cleaning, and the loads imposed by other children, a husband, and maybe parents. When a woman works at home she has no rest or meal breaks; if she works outside the home as well housework is often done in the evenings and at weekends.

Outside the home three million women work in offices, two million in hotels and shops, and one million in the health service or education; another four million work in a wide range of jobs, though few women in this country do the very heavy jobs that are done by women in the United States and the Soviet Union, for example. Indeed, in this country under the Mines Act 1889 women are not allowed to work down mines as they are in the United States. Many of the posts are part time so, though the activity may be great, the number of hours spent are fewer.

Specific hazards at work

> ### Chemical hazards in pregnancy
> - Metals—for example, lead, mercury, copper
> - Gases—for example, carbon monoxide
> - Passive smoking
> - Insecticides
> - Herbicides
> - Solvents—for example, carbon tetrachloride
> - Drugs during their manufacture
> - Disinfecting agents—for example, ethylene oxide

> ### Physical hazards in pregnancy
> - Noise
> - Vibration
> - Heat
> - Humidity
> - Repetitive muscular work—for example, at visual display units
> - Lifting heavy loads
> - Dust
> - Ionising radiation—for example, x rays

Most women are aware of specific hazards in their workplace. These are most important in very early pregnancy, when an influence may be teratogenic should the insult occur at a specific time in embryogenesis. The same stimulus acting later in pregnancy might restrict growth, causing intrauterine growth retardation.

Chemical hazards

Over 25 000 individual chemicals are used in industry, with a further 2000 compounds being added each year. It is impossible to test all of them on pregnant animals, and much of the evidence about safety depends on retrospective reports of damage to humans. The number of chemicals that are proved to be teratogenic are few.

If a woman is worried about chemicals in her workplace and consults her family doctor he would do well to discuss the problem with a health and safety officer or trade union official. If there is no help there the best reference source is the local or central office of the Health and Safety Executive. Any woman who thinks that she is working with a toxic hazard should discuss this well before pregnancy for it is often too late to start making arrangements in early pregnancy. There are special codes of practice for certain toxic chemicals which safeguard pregnant women and their unborn children. The employer should offer alternative work with no loss of pay or benefits. Toxic chemicals can still enter the mother's body after childbirth and be excreted in milk, so a lactating mother also should take precautions against toxic chemicals.

Many chemicals have been blamed at some time for affecting an early embryo. This makes big news but when, a few years later, the reports are refuted it is not newsworthy and often not reported in newspapers.

Physical hazards

At specific times in embryogenesis physical hazards can cause abnormalities. x Rays are a risk in early pregnancy, particularly if used for intravenous urography or barium studies of the intestine during the first weeks of pregnancy as multiple exposures are required. It is wise always to ask about the last menstrual period, contraceptive practices, and the possibility of pregnancy specifically before any x ray examinations are performed in women of childbearing age. The 10 day rule (whereby no

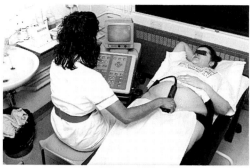

Use of ultrasound for screening.

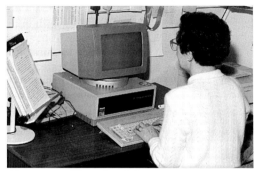

About two million visual display units are used in the United Kingdom.

Biological hazards in pregnancy

- Contact in crowded places—for example, in travelling to work
- Contact with higher risk group—for example, schoolchildren
- Food preparation
- Waterborne infections
- Arrival contacts

woman is exposed to x rays within 10 days of the next menstrual period) has now lapsed in most hospitals but inquiry should be made.

The risks of x rays in a well managed therapeutic radiation department are probably low, but some women work with radioisotopes in laboratories. The Health and Safety Executive has laid down standards that women should follow. Less well regulated are the x ray machines used for security checks in many large firms. There is probably little risk to a visitor passing once through the system, but the people who work the equipment might be exposed to repeated radiation, which should be checked.

Ultrasound is used widely in industry and at the dosage used is probably safe. Certainly, diagnostic ultrasound used in medicine has low energy and is pulsatile; the risk of cell damage or vacuolation that occurs with high energy ultrasound probably does not exist with this common use. There is no epidemiological evidence of ultrasound associated abnormalities: some 50 million women have been exposed to ultrasound in early pregnancy, yet no pattern of problems has yet been shown.

Another physical hazard which caused a recent scare was the use of visual display units (VDU). There are about 14 million such machines in use in the United States and about two million in the United Kingdom. About 10 years ago small groups of women working with visual display units were shown to have a high rate of pregnancy wastage. These were small clusters, and the measured outcomes were often a mixture of miscarriage, congenital abnormality, and stillbirth. More recent studies show no increased risk due to the use of such units, and a wide ranging review concluded, "At present it seems reasonable to conclude that pregnancy will not be harmed by using the VDU. Statements on the contrary are not soundly based."[1]

Biological hazards

Women who work in microbiological laboratories may be handling toxic materials, but usage is usually well regulated for all workers in or out of pregnancy. Animal workers may be at increased risk, and there have been reports of abortion after handling ewes at lambing because of the passage of ovine chlamydia.

Probably the most commonly transmitted infection affecting the fetus is German measles. Epidemics occur among young children, and so teachers who are constantly in contact with them are at risk. All young women entering teaching should have their serum rubella antibody titre checked; if they are found to be seronegative they should be vaccinated.

Non-specific hazards

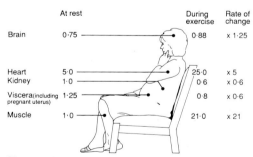

Changes in blood flow (l/min) in pregnancy.

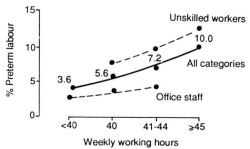

Weekly working hours and rate of preterm labour.

As well as specified toxins, various physiological changes of pregnancy in the mother might affect the embryo deleteriously. During strenuous exercise the blood supply to the non-skeletal parts of the body are reduced, including the kidneys, intestines, and uterus; the blood supply to the leg muscles can be increased 20-fold and that to the uterus halved. Hence in hard physical work, as occurs in agriculture, there may be some diminution of uterine blood flow, but this is unlikely with ordinary work. Similarly, stress can reduce blood flow to the uterus if the degree of agitation is high enough; if a woman is working inside her own limits there probably will be no problem.

Environmental factors at work that induce boredom and fatigue were found to have long term effects on pregnant women in a French study.[2] Women in industrial and agricultural jobs were compared with those working in offices. Multivariant analyses of the repetitive nature of the work, the physical effort required, the boredom of the work, standing, and the effect of background noise showed an increased proportion of preterm deliveries when these factors were high, and this might be important in women who have previously had preterm labours.

A recent British study found no effect of work on birth weight.[3] Infants born to women in full time employment had no significant differences from those born to women who were not in paid work. Data on hours of work, energy expenditure, and posture were collected at 17, 28, and 36 weeks, and these too had no discernible association with birth weight.

Work in pregnancy

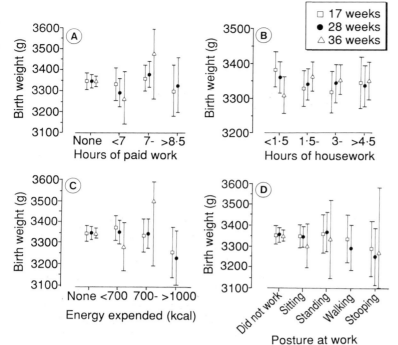

Birth weight and work. An antenatal population was sampled at 17, 28, and 36 weeks of gestation.[2]

Travel to work

If a woman has paid work outside the home she has to get there. If travelling entails a short walk in the morning and evening it can be enjoyable, but most women live in large towns with an unpleasant 30-90 minutes of travel at the beginning and end of the day. There is noise, heat, fatigue, and, in some cases, other people's tobacco. Travel is stressful in crowded, unpleasant conditions. Studies in Spain showed that the likelihood of preterm labour increases with the duration of stressful public travel the woman has to suffer.[4] It may be wise for a woman contemplating pregnancy to arrange to work flexible hours if her work is in a big city. The employer could then perhaps allow her to arrive a little before or after the rush hour, with time being made up in other ways.

Conclusions

> Pregnant women in jobs with no toxic risk need not be deterred from working for as long as they wish

More women work during pregnancy and want to continue for longer. Pregnancy is a normal event and, generally speaking, most jobs cause no increased hazard to the mother or baby. A woman should, however, be warned that if any complications arise she must be able to leave work easily. If there is flexibility and the job is not one entailing a high risk from toxic agents most women can continue working for as long as they wish in pregnancy.

The form MATB1 has Crown copyright and is reproduced by permission of the Controller of Her Majesty's Stationery Office. The figure showing weekly working hours and rate of preterm labour is reproduced by permission of the Macmillan Press from *Pregnant Women at Work* edited by G Chamberlain.

1 Blackwell R, Chang A. Video display terminals and pregnancy. *Br J Obstet Gynaecol* 1988;**95**:446-53.
2 Mamelle N, Laumon B. Occupational fatigue and preterm birth. In: Chamberlain G, ed. *Pregnant women at work*. London: Royal Society of Medicine, 1984:105-16.
3 Rabkin CS, Anderson HR, Bland JM, Brooke OG, Peacock JL, Chamberlain G. Maternal activity and birthweight. *Am J Epidemiol* 1990;**131**:522-31.
4 Rodrigues-Escudero R, Belanstegreguria A, Gutierrez-Martinez S. Perinatal complications of work and pregnancy. *An Esp Pediatr* 1980;**13**:465-76.

Recommended reading

Chamberlain G, ed. *Pregnant women at work*. London: Royal Society of Medicine, 1984.

VAGINAL BLEEDING IN EARLY PREGNANCY

Bleeding drives patients to their general practitioner swiftly. Vaginal bleeding in pregnancy makes the woman think that she may be miscarrying, so this brings her even more promptly; the practitioner thence has the opportunity to diagnose the cause and start management.

Bleeding has four known causes in early pregnancy (box). In addition, bleeding occurs for no apparent reason in a large number of cases. In early pregnancy such cases are commonly categorised as threatened miscarriage, but this is fudging the issue for in many cases the conceptus and its future placental system are not involved; doctors should be honest and say that they do not know the cause.

Causes of bleeding

- Abortion or miscarriage
- Ectopic pregnancy
- Trophoblast disease
- Lesions of the cervix or vagina

Miscarriage or abortion

The terms miscarriage and abortion are almost synonymous, but miscarriage is a softer word used for the spontaneous event.

Threatened miscarriage—Women bleed a little from the vagina during a threatened miscarriage but there is little abdominal pain. The uterus is enlarged and the cervix closed. Pregnancy may proceed.

Incomplete miscarriage—Abortion is inevitable and the cervical os is open in an incomplete miscarriage. Blood loss is often great and lower abdominal cramping pains accompany the uterine contractions. Some products of conception and clots may be passed but much decidua is retained and so the abortion is incomplete.

Complete miscarriage—The cervical os is open and the uterus completely expels its contents in a complete miscarriage. Such miscarriages are more likely after 16 weeks of pregnancy than earlier, when they are mostly incomplete.

Septic abortion follows the ascent of organisms from the vagina into the uterus, often after an incomplete or induced abortion under non-sterile conditions. As well as heavy bleeding and pain, the woman commonly has a fever and may develop signs of endotoxic shock. The commonest organisms are *Escherichia coli* and *Streptococcus faecalis*.

Types of miscarriage

- Threatened miscarriage
- Inevitable miscarriage
  Complete
  Incomplete
- Missed abortion
- Recurrent miscarriage
- Criminal abortion
- Septic abortion
- Therapeutic abortion

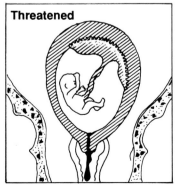 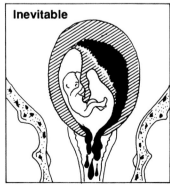 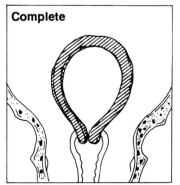 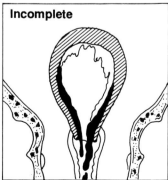

In a threatened abortion the cervix is still closed and there is not much bleeding; in an inevitable miscarriage the cervix has started to open and the membranes often have ruptured. There is usually more bleeding.

A complete miscarriage means that the uterus is empty of clot and decidua, whereas in an incomplete miscarriage the embryo has been passed vaginally but some part of the membrane or decidua is retained. There may also be clots.

Vaginal bleeding in early pregnancy

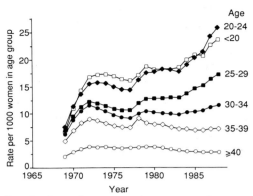

Terminations of pregnancy by age group in England and Wales, 1968-88. More operations are performed outside the NHS, some being done through charity clinics.

Missed abortion—The embryo dies and is absorbed but the uterus does not expel the decidua and sac of membranes in a missed abortion. The woman feels a dull weight in the pelvis and the uterus stops enlarging. Old blood is passed as a brown, watery discharge. This condition is diagnosed more frequently now that ultrasonography is used in very early pregnancy.

Recurrent abortion is diagnosed when a woman has three or more spontaneous miscarriages. Such women deserve gynaecological and immunological investigation; many gynaecologists start investigations after two consecutive miscarriages in women over 35.

Therapeutic abortion is now common in Britain, with over 170 000 women in England and Wales having such abortions each year. Usually the general practitioner knows but occasionally the woman has bypassed him, presenting only after the event with vaginal bleeding, an open cervix, and some abdominal pain. This means that decidua or blood clot is left and needs the same attention as does any other incomplete miscarriage.

Causes

Embryonic abnormalities—Chromosomal abnormalities are common, arising from a change in the nucleus of either gamete or a spontaneous mutation inside the fertilised oocyte. At the time of fertilisation splitting and rejoining of genetic material may be imperfect. Such changes are not usually recurrent, and parents should be told this.

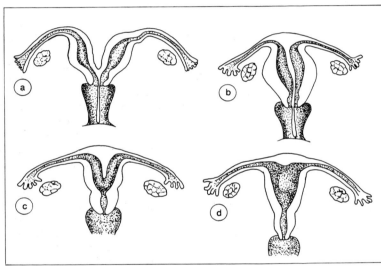

Congenital abnormalities of the uterus caused by non-absorption of the septum during the fusion of the two Müllerian ducts. (*a*) Complete double uterus, double cervix, and vaginal septum. (*b*) Double uterine cavity within a single body; the cervix and the vagina has a septum. (*c*) A subseptate uterus in which the septum does not reach down to the cervix. (*d*) Arcuate uterus with a dimple on top of the single uterus with a single cervix.

Immunological rejection—The fetus is genetically foreign to the mother and yet most fetuses are not rejected. In many cases blocking antibodies that inhibit the cell mediated rejection of the embryo are stimulated by antigens from the trophoblast. If a couple share more HLA antigens than usual, the trophoblast may not stimulate production of these maternal blocking antibodies and embryonic tissue will be rejected. Up to 30% of spontaneous miscarriages have been attributed to this reason. If there are recurrent miscarriages both sets of antigens should be checked.

Uterine abnormalities—The uterus is formed during embryonic development from two tubes fusing together to make a common cavity. Occasionally various degrees of non-absorption in the midline septum occur, leaving either two cavities or a cavity partly divided by a septum down the middle. The blood supply to this median structure is usually poor and implantation of an embryo here may be followed by miscarriage.

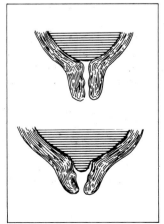

Cervical incompetence.

Cervical incompetence—The cervix may have some weakness—either congenital or acquired after a previous harsh dilatation—which could be associated with a spontaneous miscarriage in the mid-trimester (13-27 weeks). The unsupported membranes bulge into the cervical canal through the internal os and rupture early, which causes the abortive process. The incompetence may be diagnosed before pregnancy by a hysterogram (a radiological examination of the uterine cavity) or in pregnancy by ultrasonography. Most treatment, however, is started when there is a history of mid-trimester miscarriage, particularly if the membranes ruptured before any uterine contractions occurred.

Maternal disease is unlikely to be a major cause of miscarriage in the United Kingdom, but hypertension and renal disease are still associated with higher rates of miscarriage in later pregnancy. Maternal infections can affect the fetus, particularly rubella, toxoplasmosis, cytomegalic inclusion disease, and listeriosis. Severe maternal malnutrition is most unusual in this country, though it can still occur in developing countries. Deficiency of individual vitamins (such as vitamin E) is extraordinarily rare in the mixed diet of this country, and there is no evidence of its being a substantial cause of miscarriage in women.

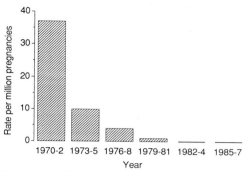

The number of deaths reported after illegal abortion is reducing rapidly in England and Wales. Death used to be mostly from sepsis or from renal or hepatic failure.

Endocrine imbalance—Diabetes and thyroid hyperfunction used to be associated with increased risks of spontaneous miscarriage. If diagnosed, both are now usually well treated and women have a good hormone balance. An insufficiency of progesterone from the corpus luteum used to be regarded as a cause of miscarriage. This is hard to prove, and most randomised trials using progestogens in early pregnancy have failed to show an improvement. If, however, the woman has faith in this treatment and had a previous successful pregnancy taking it, the practitioner would do well to treat the psyche as well as the soma and prescribe a progestogen.

Criminal abortion is now much less common in Britain but still occurs in other countries and in populations derived from those countries. Although infection has been introduced, only rarely do criminal abortionists leave signs that can be spotted in the genital tract and so the woman is often treated for an incomplete or septic miscarriage.

Presentation

A woman who is miscarrying usually presents with vaginal bleeding and may have some low abdominal pain. The bleeding is slight in a threatened miscarriage, greater amounts being present with an inevitable miscarriage. Pain with uterine contractions may be compared with dysmenorrhoea. The degree of shock usually relates to the amount of blood loss from the body.

The differential diagnosis includes ectopic pregnancy and salpingitis.

Management

Threatened miscarriage—A woman with a threatened miscarriage is best removed from an active environment. If the practitioner tells her to go to bed to rest for 48 hours she may feel happier but there is no real evidence that bedrest makes any difference to the incidence of miscarriage. Some 5% of women who deliver safely report a threatened miscarriage in the same pregnancy; the effectiveness of specific treatments is difficult to assess. The avoidance of sexual intercourse is probably sensible as it might act as a local stimulus.

Inevitable miscarriage—If events progress to an inevitable miscarriage the woman needs to be admitted to hospital; an oxytocic agent might be given if the bleeding is excessive and a flying squad may be needed. After admission an evacuation will be performed under general anaesthesia.

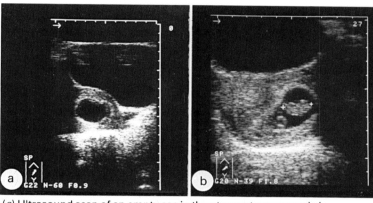

(*a*) Ultrasound scan of an empty sac in the uterus at seven weeks' gestation. This woman had a missed abortion, the embryo having been resorbed. (*b*) Ultrasound scan of a continuing pregnancy at just over seven weeks; fetal tissue is easily seen between the arrows.

Treatment of severe septic abortion

- **Hypovolaemia**
  Monitor—Blood pressure
           Central venous pressure
           Cardiac output
           Renal output
  Treatment—Intravenous rehydration and maintenance
- **Infection**
  Identify organisms
  Treatment—Systemic
           Antibodies
      —Local
           Evacuate uterus (dilatation and curettage)
           ? Remove uterus (hysterectomy)
- **Coagulation abnormalities**
- **Respiratory system**
  Monitor—Blood gases
  Treatment—Oxygen
           ? Ventilate
- **Anaemia and white cell deficiencies**

Complete abortion is unusual; the practitioner may see the sac containing the embryo and feel that this is complete. He would do well to remember, however, that a large amount of decidua is left behind and an evacuation may prevent the woman having a haemorrhage or infection a week or so later.

Missed abortion is usually diagnosed from the woman's symptoms of a brown discharge and a heavy, dull feeling in the pelvis; the finding of no embryonic tissue inside the gestation sac on ultrasonography confirms the diagnosis. It is wise to evacuate the uterus under anaesthesia, but this may occur on the next elective operating list unless bleeding is heavy.

Septic abortion may require the full management of severe sepsis. Endocervical swabs should be sent to the laboratory and treatment with a broad spectrum antibiotic started immediately afterwards. Central venous pressure measurement and intravenous rehydration will be required; the urinary output should be watched carefully. Evidence of disseminated intravascular coagulopathy should be assessed and the uterus evacuated once a reasonable tissue concentration of antibiotics has been achieved.

Recurrent abortion—The management of recurrent abortion is outside the scope of this series. It requires sympathetic handling by both general practitioners and specialists.

Vaginal bleeding in early pregnancy
Ectopic pregnancy

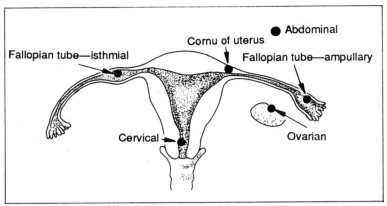

Possible sites for ectopic pregnancy.

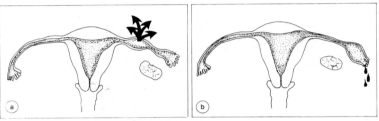

The most common ectopic pregnancies are in the fallopian tube. Those at the medial end rupture (*a*), those at the lateral end leak (*b*).

Symptoms and signs of ectopic pregnancy

	Unruptured	Ruptured
Symptoms	Gradual onset	Sudden onset
	Dull ache over days	Severe pain over minutes
Signs	No shock	Commonly shock
	Vague suprapubic tenderness	Rigid abdomen with rebound tenderness
	No great cervical tenderness	Extreme tenderness on cervical movement
	Vague mass often felt	Too tender to palpate

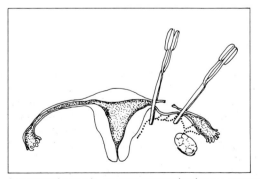

A ruptured ectopic pregnancy nearly always means excision of the damaged tissue. This is done by clamping off the tube on either side as the blood supply is usually in the mesenteric border of the tube in the broad ligament.

An ectopic pregnancy is one that implants and develops outside the uterine cavity. The sites are shown in the figure, but most (96%) are in the fallopian tube.

Causes

Anything that slows the passage of the fertilised oocyte down the fallopian tube can cause a tubal ectopic pregnancy. Previous tubal infection, an intrauterine device in place, and late fertilisation are quoted causes, but in most ectopic pregnancies no cause is found.

Presentation

A tubal ectopic pregnancy may either rupture through the wall (more common with isthmial and cornual implantations) or leak a little blood from the lateral end of the fallopian tube (with ampullary or fimbrial implantations). After a variable number of weeks of amenorrhoea vaginal bleeding can occur.

With rupture there is a brisk peritoneal reaction and the woman may fall to the ground as though kicked in the stomach. She quickly becomes very shocked. The abdomen is tender with guarding and rebound tenderness, and vaginal examination causes intense pain on touching the cervix.

A more gradual leak causes irritation of the pouch of Douglas. The woman goes to her doctor complaining of vague, low abdominal pain, sometimes with vaginal bleeding occurring after the pain. The abdomen may be uncomfortable in the suprapubic area, and a very gentle vaginal assessment may show a tenderness in the pouch of Douglas or in the adnexa on one side.

The differential diagnosis includes an abortion or any other cause for a sudden release of blood into the peritoneal cavity, such as a bleeding vessel over an ovarian cyst. Inflammatory conditions such as appendicitis may mimic a leaking ectopic pregnancy. Ectopic pregnancy should always be considered in any cases of lower abdominal pain for an unruptured ectopic pregnancy, leaking a little blood over the course of some days, is hard to diagnose.

Management

The management of a woman with a ruptured ectopic pregnancy is straightforward. She should go to hospital immediately, if necessary accompanied by her general practitioner. Intravenous treatment may be required in the home, and in severe cases a flying squad may be required. Once in the hospital surgery should be immediate and the area bleeding should be clamped off. The surgeon may have to remove the whole fallopian tube, but this would depend on how much damage has occurred. If some part of the tube can be left behind it is psychologically helpful to the woman. There is a small risk of a second ectopic pregnancy developing in the stump but there is also the possibility of reparative surgery later. This is very important when a woman has had two ectopic pregnancies and a fallopian tube has already been removed.

A leaking tubal pregnancy is harder to diagnose, such cases being usually referred to outpatient departments in a more leisurely fashion. If the diagnosis is suspected laparoscopy is the best test; ultrasonography is not exclusive, although fluid in the pouch of Douglas and no intrauterine pregnancy in a woman with 6-8 weeks' amenorrhoea is highly suggestive. At laparoscopy the swollen area of the tube can usually be seen and little blood may come from the lateral end. Conventional surgeons would remove the affected area of the tube at a laparotomy, but now many gynaecologists treat non-ruptured ectopic pregnancies through a laparoscope. Embryo death can be ensured by injection, or a salpingostomy can be performed using laparoscopy directed cutting and diathermy equipment when the conceptus and decidua are sucked out; the results of such minimalist surgery are as good as those of more conservative surgery, with the time spent in hospital and the emotional effects on the woman's life being much reduced.

> Any woman treated for an ectopic pregnancy should be warned of the increased chances of a recurrence on the other side. The increased risk is said to be seven times above background

Gestational trophoblastic disease

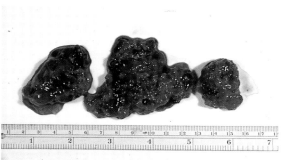 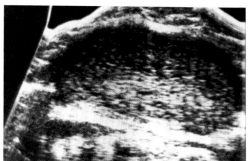

Left: Hydatidiform mole. The bunch of vesicles rapidly expands the uterine cavity. Right: A hydatidiform mole may be diagnosed readily on ultrasonography, the sound waves being reflected off the vesicles to give a picture of soap bubble foam. With early ultrasound equipment, however, hydatidiform moles looked like a snowstorm.

Human chorionic gonadotrophin values are much higher in women with a hydatidiform mole than in women with a normal pregnancy (note the log scale).

Causes

Chromosomal changes in the fertilised oocyte lead to degeneration of the stem blood vessels in the villi in very early pregnancy, so producing a vast overgrowth of vesicles inside the uterus. This is a hydatidiform mole, and commonly no embryo is found. It is usually benign but in less than 10% of cases it develops into an invasive mole or even a gestational choriocarcinoma.

Although rare in the United Kingdom (0·6 per 1000 pregnancies), hydatidiform moles and their malignant sequelae seem to be reported more commonly in other parts of the world such as in the Pacific region (2·0 per 1000 pregnancies).

Presentation

A woman with a mole will bleed, sometimes heavily, after eight weeks of gestation. She is often unwell with signs of anaemia and excessive vomiting. Proteinuric hypertension can occur as early as eight weeks. After 12 weeks of gestation the uterus often feels much bigger than expected for dates but no fetal parts can be felt or fetal heart heard. Occasionally the woman may pass vesicles through the vagina; this is diagnostic but rarely occurs.

Moles are diagnosed either from an excessively high estimation of human chorionic gonadotrophin in the urine or by ultrasonography, when a characteristic picture is seen.

The differential diagnosis must include twins with a threatened miscarriage, but ultrasonography, which should be readily available to most general practitioners, gives the answer immediately.

Vaginal bleeding in early pregnancy

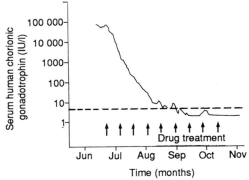

After evacuation of a hydatidiform mole the human chorionic gonadotrophin concentration remains high. Methotrexate and folinic acid were given on nine occasions, the treatment being associated with a reduction in hormone concentration.

Management

Once diagnosed a mole should be evacuated quickly. The woman should be admitted to hospital and a suction curettage performed under anaesthesia with the protection of an oxytocin drip. All tissue is sent to the laboratory for examination of its neoplastic potential.

After a mole all women should be registered for follow up at one of the supraregional trophoblast disease centres, where human chorionic gonadotrophin concentrations in urine or blood can be measured. If these are high at six weeks chemotherapy is recommended to prevent subsequent malignancy.

Other causes of vaginal bleeding

Lesions of the cervix or vagina may cause bleeding in early pregnancy

Bleeding may come from local problems in the vagina or cervix.

- Cervical erosion is common in pregnancy; bleeding is not profuse
- Vaginal or cervical infections with monilia can cause mild bleeding
- Adenomas and polyps of the cervix become more pronounced during pregnancy. They may bleed on stimulation
- Carcinoma of the cervix is rare but important in women of childbearing age. It may cause bleeding on stimulation and examination with a speculum reveals the cause. If there is any doubt a biopsy must be performed under anaesthesia even when a woman is pregnant
- A general maternal disease such as blood dysplasia, von Willebrand's disease, or leukaemia may cause symptoms in rare cases.

I thank Dr Rashmi Patel for the ultrasound pictures. The figure showing treatment of a hydatidiform mole is reproduced by permission of Churchill Livingstone from *Obstetrics*, edited by A Turnbull and G Chamberlain.

MEDICAL PROBLEMS IN PREGNANCY—I

Problem diseases in pregnancy
- Heart disease
- Diabetes
- Thyroid disease
- Epilepsy
- Jaundice
- Anaemia
- Haemoglobinopathies
- Urinary tract infection
- Psychiatric changes and diseases

Pregnant women are usually young and fit. They rarely have chronic medical conditions, but when they do those in charge of antenatal care need to consider how the disease might affect pregnancy and how pregnancy might affect the disease.

Heart disease

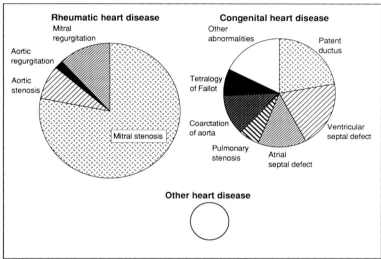

Main causes of heart disease in pregnancy, the area of the circle reflecting the proportional frequency. Other causes of heart disease include thyrotoxicosis and coronary artery disease.

Mitral stenosis. Narrowing of the mitral valve can lead to back pressure in the pulmonary circulation in late pregnancy and just after delivery.

Most heart disease in women of childbearing age is rheumatic in origin despite the recent great reduction in the prevalence of rheumatic fever. Better living conditions and the more prompt treatment of streptococcal sore throats with antibiotics in childhood have reduced rheumatic damage to the heart valves and myocardium. An increasing proportion of pregnant women have congenital heart lesions that have been treated previously.

Pregnancy puts an increased load on the cardiovascular system. More blood has to be circulated so that cardiac output increases by up to 40% by mid-pregnancy, staying steady until labour, when it increases further. This increased cardiac work cannot be done as effectively by a damaged heart; if the heart is compromised a woman would be wise to avoid other increased loads that might precipitate cardiac failure. The most frequently encountered are:

- Household work
- Paid work outside the home
- Care of other family members
- Pre-eclampsia
- Anaemia

- Recrudescence of rheumatic fever
- Respiratory infection
- Urinary infection
- Bacterial endocarditis.

Care should be taken just after delivery: with a uterine contraction up to a litre of blood can be shunted from the uterine into the general venous system.

The commonest single cardiac lesion found in women of this age group is rheumatic mitral stenosis, sometimes accompanied by the after effects of rheumatic myocarditis. The commonest complication of overload is pulmonary oedema in late pregnancy or immediately after delivery. Right sided cardiac failure may occur but is less common.

Cardiomyopathy of pregnancy occurs mostly post partum but occasionally in late pregnancy. There is no obvious predisposing cause; the heart is greatly distorted, leading to right sided cardiac failure.

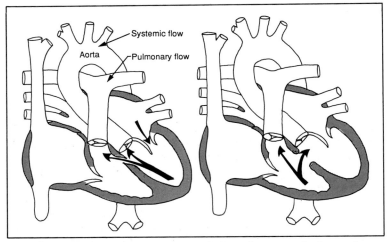

Eisenmenger's syndrome. The right to left shunt that occurs in the syndrome in pregnancy can rapidly precipitate congestive heart failure.

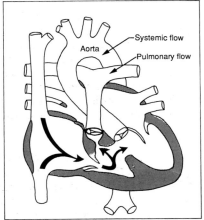

Tetralogy of Fallot. If the prepulmonary stenosis is severe right to left shunting occurs.

Modified New York Heart Association's classification of cardiac functional capacity

	Symptoms of cardiac insufficiency	Limitation of activities
I	None	None
II	Only after exercise	With moderate exercise
III	After any activity	With ordinary activities
IV	At rest	Unable to perform any physical activities

The most serious of the congenital lesions in pregnancy are those accompanied by shunts.

● Women with Eisenmenger's syndrome do particularly badly in pregnancy, especially those with severe pulmonary hypertension, which leads to a right to left shunt

● Tetralogy of Fallot has a lower risk of cardiac failure because there is less resistance at the pulmonary valve regulating right ventricular outflow.

Other congenital abnormalities found in pregnancy are:

● Coarctation of the aorta, which has usually been detected beforehand and, if repaired, results in little increased danger in pregnancy.

The risk of a fetus having congenital heart disease is increased if the mother has the same problem; it ranges from 1:4 in tetralogy of Fallot to 1:15 in atrial septal defects

● Artificial heart valves, which are now present in an increasing number of women who become pregnant. Commonly they are manmade replacements of the mitral or aortic valve; affected women receive anticoagulant treatment and should continue to do so. Warfarin is the commonest agent and despite the theoretical risk of teratogenesis in early pregnancy and fetal bleeding later it is still the most effective anticoagulant for patients with artificial valves. It is still widely used and should continue to be taken until the very end of pregnancy, when it may be replaced two or three weeks before the expected date of delivery by heparin.

Management

Most women with heart disease who are of childbearing age are known to their family practitioner. He or she should ensure that they go for antenatal care at a centre where a cardiologist works alongside an obstetrician, ideally at a combined cardiac antenatal clinic.

Early assessment should be made of the severity of the disease, paying attention to the features that may worsen the prognosis: the woman's age, the severity of the lesion, the type of lesion, and the degree of decompensation (exercise tolerance). Rest should be encouraged during pregnancy and extra physical loads avoided. Labour should be booked at a consultant unit with an interested cardiologist involved.

Care should be taken to avoid the development of acute bacterial endocarditis by ensuring that the woman is given antibiotics when she has any infection or is at potential risk of developing an infection—for example, when having a tooth extracted. This precaution is more important for congenital lesions of the heart than for rheumatic lesions.

The prognosis for a woman with heart disease in pregnancy is now greatly improved. It used inevitably to be associated with deterioration of the heart condition, but now, with proper care, this is not so.

Diabetes

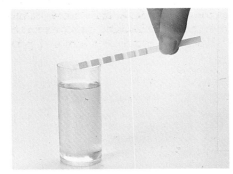

Dipstick testing of urine.

Diabetes is a metabolic disease found in about 1% of women of childbearing age. In addition, another 1% or 2% of women will develop gestational diabetes during the course of their pregnancy; the incidence is higher in older than younger women. Glycosuria (checked by dipstick testing) is even more common than this, occurring at some time in pregnancy in up to 15% of women.

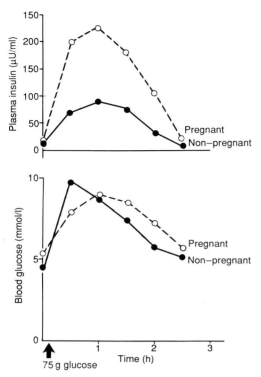

Plasma insulin and blood glucose response to oral glucose (75 g) in pregnant and non-pregnant women.

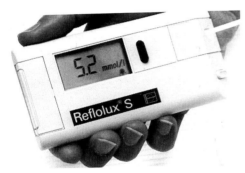

Blood glucose concentration meter for home use.

Vaginal delivery in diabetic mothers

Good prognostic features
- Primigravida <30
- Multigravida with good obstetric history
- Estimated fetal weight <3500 g
- Well engaged cephalic presentation
- Stable diabetic control

Bad prognostic features
- Primigravida >30
- Multigravida with poor obstetric history
- Large fetus (>3500 g)
- Non-engageable head or breech presentation
- Unstable diabetes

Established insulin dependent diabetes

Four fifths of women with diabetes are known to the practitioner before they become pregnant. All diabetic women of reproductive age should be using effective contraception and be encouraged to attend a pre-pregnancy clinic. Tight control of diabetes before and in early pregnancy reduces the incidence of congenital anomalies.

Antenatal care is best performed by an obstetrician and a diabetic physician at a combined diabetic antenatal clinic. The general practitioner must be kept well informed of changes in management of the diabetes during pregnancy, as between antenatal clinic visits the woman will depend on her family practitioner for continuity of care. Detailed ultrasonography to exclude congenital abnormalities and to monitor growth is vital.

Pregnancy makes the control of diabetes more difficult. Virtually all diabetic women require an increase in their insulin dosage during pregnancy and requirements may vary so that tighter control is required. Glucose concentrations in blood rather than urine should be used to judge insulin dosage. This is often done at home with sticks and a glucose meter. Hospital admission for control of glucose concentration is rarely needed in established diabetes. Immediately after delivery diabetic women return swiftly to their previous insulin requirements so they should be watched carefully.

Diabetic women with proliferative retinopathy should be offered laser coagulation before embarking on pregnancy. Proliferative retinopathy that arises or worsens during the first trimester should, however, no longer be seen as a reason for termination, and laser treatment is safe and effective in pregnancy. Diabetic vascular complications almost never occur in women of reproductive age. Renal complications are rare but require careful management by the hospital team.

Management—Twice daily regimens of short and medium acting insulin may be effective in the first half of pregnancy, but preprandial soluble insulin with a long acting insulin in the evening is often needed later. Hypertension and infection are indications for admitting the woman to hospital. Most obstetricians no longer admit women routinely at 32 weeks if there are no complications, allowing pregnancy to proceed to near term. At about 38 weeks the obstetric situation is assessed. If there are good prognostic factors a vaginal delivery will be attempted, but if any of the high risk features are present an elective caesarean section is usually performed (box).

Diabetes controlled by oral hypoglycaemic agents

Generally women with diabetes controlled by oral hypoglycaemic agents have a safer pregnancy; their condition is easier to maintain when their oral treatment is substituted by low dose soluble insulin. Such women are then monitored in the same way as women with established insulin dependent diabetes.

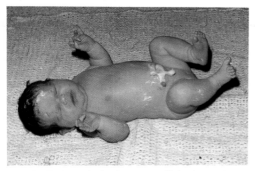

A typically large baby born to a diabetic mother.

Gestational diabetes

Gestational diabetes is diagnosed when a woman develops abnormal glucose tolerance for the first time in pregnancy; a number of women will remain diabetic after the pregnancy. Traditionally, screening has been by performing glucose tolerance tests on all women who are themselves overweight (usually >100 kg), have given birth to a big baby (usually >4500 g), have had an unexplained stillbirth, or have a first degree relative with insulin dependent diabetes. Additionally, glucose tolerance tests have been performed on women who have glycosuria once before 20 weeks' gestation or twice thereafter. Such criteria lead to a very low rate of positive test results. Currently, many hospitals will perform a random blood glucose test at 28-34 weeks, interpreting the result in relation to the timing of the last meal. Women with high values will then have a glucose tolerance test or have blood glucose concentrations measured serially (preprandial and postprandial tests three times a day) to determine whether they are glucose intolerant.

Women with gestational diabetes do not have an increased rate of babies with congenital abnormalities but the babies are at risk of being large. There is no consensus on treatment, which ranges from controlling dietary intake to insulin treatment and dietary control. Such women usually have labour induced at term and are at risk of having long labours and shoulder dystocia.

After delivery insulin should be stopped; all affected women should have a glucose tolerance test at six weeks. About 15-20% of such women will develop non-insulin dependent diabetes (type II) in later life but this proportion rises to 70% among those who are obese.

Thyroid disease

Effect of thyrotoxicosis and pregnancy on some thyroid function tests

	Thyrotoxicosis	Pregnancy
Triiodothyronine:		
Free	Increased	No change
Protein bound	Increased	Increased
Thyroxine:		
Free	Increased	No change
Protein bound	Increased	Increased
Thyroxine binding globulin	No change	Increased

Hyperthyroidism

Women who are already hyperthyroid are usually receiving treatment, which may have to be continued throughout pregnancy. However, some of these women may be nearing the end of a 12-18 month course of antithyroid treatment and others find that their hyperthyroidism ameliorates in the last weeks of pregnancy. In such cases withdrawal of antithyroid drugs may reduce the severity of fetal goitre. These women should be tested for the presence of thyroid antibodies of the IgG class (long acting thyroid stimulator and thyroid receptor antibodies) as they cross the placenta and cause neonatal thyrotoxicosis when present in high titres. Thyroid crises (storm crises) are now rare in pregnancy and the immediate puerperium. They are best treated with iodine, which works quicker than β blockade and carbimazole. Operation on the thyroid is rarely indicated in pregnancy but is safe in the midtrimester.

Hypothyroidism

Hypothyroid women are commonly anovular. If they are receiving adequate replacement treatment, however, they ovulate as normal. Such treatment should be continued and may need to be increased during pregnancy.

Epilepsy

Therapeutic concentrations of anticonvulsants in blood

	mg/l
Phenytoin	10-12
Phenobarbitone	15-40
Carbamazepine	4-12
Primidone	5-12
Ethosuximide	4-100

An epileptic woman will often consult her family practitioner before becoming pregnant as she may have heard of the potential hazards of antiepileptic drugs. Before making any recommendations the general practitioner would be wise to consult a neurologist about each individual patient. Though most antiepileptic drugs have teratogenic properties to different extents, epileptic women have an inbuilt increased risk of having babies with malformations even without treatment. This risk and the risks to the embryo if the woman has a series of convulsions when anticonvulsant treatment is withdrawn in early pregnancy should be carefully balanced.

Generally, the woman may stop or modify treatment after full consultation when she has not had a recent fit. If she needs treatment the same dose must be continued; phenytoin treatment seems to be associated with a lower risk of fetal neural tube defects and might be substituted.

Seizure frequency seems to be the same in pregnancy as outside pregnancy for most epileptic women; if the rate of fitting worsens, blood concentrations of all anticonvulsants should be checked as overdose as well as underdose may be responsible for loss of seizure control. Prophylactic folic acid (5 mg/day) should be given during pregnancy as folate absorption is changed by the antiepileptic drugs. Vitamin K should be given to all the newborn infants of such mothers for similar reasons.

Status epilepticus is unusual in a pregnant woman unless she is known to be a severe epileptic. Diazepam is the best drug of the active treatments.

> For most epileptic women the frequency of seizures is not affected by pregnancy

Jaundice

Some causes of jaundice in pregnancy

Pregnancy associated
- Cholestasis
  Raised oestrogen concentrations
- Acute fatty liver of pregnancy
- Disseminated intravascular coagulopathy
- Severe pre-eclampsia
- Excessive vomiting (hyperemesis)
- Severe septicaemia in late pregnancy

Unrelated to pregnancy
- Viral hepatitis
- Drugs
  Chlorpromazine
  Tetracycline
  Steroids
- Chronic liver disease
- Gall stones
- Chronic haemolysis

The commonest causes of jaundice in pregnancy are the various forms of hepatitis and drugs that affect the liver. Gall stones and severe pre-eclampsia may be responsible, but gall stones are rare in the age group concerned. Cholestasis in the last trimester may occur spontaneously or follow the use of steroids, fatty degeneration of the liver in the last weeks of pregnancy is very rare but can lead to liver failure. Severe pre-eclampsia may uncommonly lead to jaundice.

The results of the conventional liver function tests are not as helpful during pregnancy, and the early participation of hepatic experts in the care of a woman with jaundice during pregnancy is wise.

The table showing therapeutic concentrations of anticonvulsants is based on that by J Donaldson in *Critical Care of the Obstetric Patient*, edited by R Berkowitz, and is reproduced by permission of Churchill Livingstone. The photographs of the dipstick testing and glucose testing equipment are reproduced by permission of Boehringer Mannheim (United Kingdom).

MEDICAL PROBLEMS IN PREGNANCY—II

Anaemia

Normal haematological values in pregnancy

	Range
Total blood volume (ml)	4000-6000
Red cell volume (ml)	1500-1800
Red cell count (10^{12}/l)	4-5
White cell count (10^9/l)	10-15
Haemoglobin (g/dl)	11·0-13·5
Erythrocyte sedimentation rate (mm in the first hour)	10-60
Mean corpuscular volume (μm^3)	80-95
Mean corpuscular haemoglobin (pg)	27-32
Serum iron (μmol/l)	11-25
Total iron binding capacity (μmol/l)	40-70
Serum ferritin (μg/l)	10-200
Serum folate (μg/l)	6-9

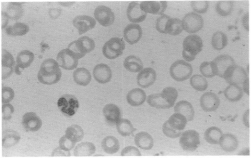

Iron deficiency anaemia.

Indices of iron deficiency anaemia

Blood film

- Red cells
  Normal size or microcytic
  Hypochromic
  Anisocytosis
  Poikilocytosis

Haematological values

- Haemoglobin ↓
- Mean corpuscular volume ↓
- Mean corpuscular haemoglobin ↓
- Serum iron ↓
- Serum ferritin ↓

A few pregnant women may have a chronic haematological condition predating pregnancy; some acquire anaemia during pregnancy as a result of dietary changes and the metabolic demands of pregnancy on maternal and fetal physiology.

Clinical anaemia is often asymptomatic in pregnancy as small falls below the widely accepted lower limit of haemoglobin concentration (11 g/dl) are rarely accompanied by symptoms. Most anaemias in Britain are detected by blood tests done routinely at antenatal clinics. Occasionally, a woman will present more quickly with symptomatic anaemia, especially in countries where malnutrition is common.

Anaemia in pregnancy is mostly due to:

- Lack of production of haemoglobin, mostly because of low concentrations of iron and other blood synthesising precursors—for example, folate

- A chronic repeated blood loss from aspirin ingestion or, overseas, hookworm infection

- Haemolysis of circulating blood cells—rarely seen in white women but common in other races.

Most anaemias detected in the United Kingdom during pregnancy are due to lack of production of haemoglobin, the haemopoietic system being unable to respond to the extra load of pregnancy because of a lack of iron and folic acid.

Iron deficiency anaemia

The haemodilution of pregnancy causes a fall in haemoglobin concentration of approximately 1-2 g/dl. Iron deficiency in pregnancy is usually due to a diet deficient in iron; in rare cases iron absorption from the intestine is faulty. In the United Kingdom this condition occurs in about 10% of women and is usually detected in mid-pregnancy by routine tests.

During pregnancy the demand for iron is increased. The total intake in pregnancy should be 700-1400 mg to allow for the increase in maternal red cell volume, fetal iron requirements, and uterine growth. Thus daily requirements rise from 2 mg a day in non-pregnant women to 3·5-4 mg a day in pregnancy. Absorption from the intestine increases in pregnancy so one 60 mg tablet a day would suffice if it was taken regularly.

If the woman has iron deficiency anaemia with a haemoglobin concentration below 11·0 g/dl a blood film will show microcytosis and hypochromia. A comparatively low haemoglobin concentration can, however, be accompanied by only slight changes in red cell indices. The mean cell haemoglobin and the serum iron concentration will be low if the iron deficiency anaemia persists. Serum ferritin concentrations are probably the best guide to the amount of iron stored in the body. The number of reticulocytes increases when the bone marrow responds to the treatment of anaemia.

Iron deficiency anaemia is best prevented by ensuring that the woman has a diet containing sufficient iron. Preferably this will entail eating foods with a higher iron content, including meat (a little liver and kidney), egg yolks, beans, peas, and dried fruits such as apricots, raisins, and prunes. High roughage foods such as wholemeal flour, bran, and muesli tend to inhibit iron absorption and should be eaten in moderation.

Dose and ferrous iron content of commonly prescribed iron tablets

	Dose (mg)	Ferrous iron content (mg)
Ferrous sulphate (dried)	200	60
Ferrous sulphate	300	60
Ferrous fumarate	200	65
Ferrous gluconate	300	35
Ferrous succinate	100	35

Parenteral iron preparations

- Iron dextran
  Complex of ferric hydroxide with dextrans of high molecular weight
  Iron content 50 mg/ml
  Intravenous or intramuscular route (check with test dose in case of anaphylaxis)
  Proprietary preparation: Imferon

- Iron sorbitol
  Complex of iron, sorbitol, and citric acid
  Iron content 50 mg/ml
  Intramuscular route only
  Proprietary preparation: Jectofer

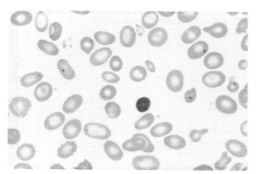

Megaloblastic anaem

Indices of megaloblastic anaemia

Blood film
- Red cells
  Normal size or macrocytic
  Normochromic
  Anisocytosis
  Poikilocytosis
  Sometimes nuclear material
- White cells
  Leucopenia
  Hypersegmentation
- Platelets
  Sometimes thrombocytopenia

Haematological values
- Haemoglobin ↓
- Mean corpuscular volume ↑ or =
- Mean corpuscular haemoglobin ↑
- Serum iron ↑
- Red cell folate ↓
- Marrow
  Megaloblastosis

In the United Kingdom supplementary iron was commonly given to all pregnant women as tablets of ferrous sulphate (200 mg), fumarate (200 mg), or succinate (100 mg), one of which will suit most women. The different preparations contain 35-60 mg of ferrous iron in each tablet and about 100 mg a day is required from food and tablets to present the intestinal mucosa with adequate ferrous ions. Many doctors now rely on the results of blood tests taken during pregnancy, giving iron only to those who are or become really anaemic, and give advice on an iron rich diet. This is a logical approach for most women in this country.

Sometimes a woman cannot take iron tablets, so if it is necessary a liquid preparation should be prescribed. If the patient is unable to take oral iron it may be given intravenously or intramuscularly, with precautions being taken against anaphylaxis. If severe anaemia (haemoglobin concentration below 8·5 g/dl) is not detected until the last four weeks of pregnancy, blood transfusion is required to cover labour as the body has not enough time to manufacture sufficient circulating haemoglobin to ward off the increased risk of blood loss at delivery. It is unsafe for any woman to approach labour with a haemoglobin concentration below 8·5 g/dl

Folate deficiency anaemia

Folate deficiency anaemia is rarer than iron deficiency anaemia in the United Kingdom. Nowadays it is usually detected from red cell indices as an anaemia with a raised mean cell volume. All tissue production requires folate for the manufacture of DNA; in pregnancy folate demands are higher from both the fetus and the increased maternal demands. As well as the increased requirements, there may be a deficiency in the diet. In developing countries this is often associated with a deficiency in other vitamins.

A woman with folate deficiency may present with symptoms of anaemia, being breathless and looking pale, and she may have other signs of poor nutrition. Haematological tests show a low haemoglobin concentration, often well below 8·0 g/dl. A blood film may show macrocytosis, but this result is inconstant. The mean cell volume is increased while the neutrophils may show multisegmentation of the nucleus. Serum iron concentration is high, but the concentration of folic acid in the red cells is low. These indices usually enable diagnosis, but occasionally aspiration of a blood marrow sample from the iliac crest is required to show megaloblastic changes.

Management—Prevention is the best management of folic acid deficiency. Foods with a high folate content are recommended such as beans, dark green leaf vegetables, legumes, yeast extracts, and fish; folate is commonly given prophylactically to most women attending for antenatal care. It is often combined with the prophylactic iron preparation so that one tablet a day contains 300-500 µg folate, which is more than enough to prevent folic acid deficiency. The theoretical fear of masking combined degeneration of the spinal cord in association with pernicious anaemia is extremely unlikely in women of reproductive age. If a woman has a proved folate deficiency anaemia she should be treated with oral folic acid 5-10 mg a day. Theoretically she may not need extra iron above that which she is already having if her iron stores are replete, but often this is not so and folate deficiency accompanies iron deficiency. Furthermore, once folate treatment has started the woman may become iron deficient rapidly. When women with very low indices are excluded, there is rarely a need to give a blood transfusion because the haemopoietic system responds swiftly when adequate folate and iron are provided, and the woman replaces her own blood cells.

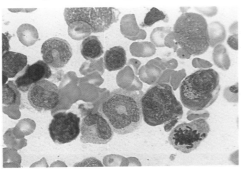

Bone marrow aspirate.

Haemoglobinopathies

Haemorrhagic anaemia

Haemorrhagic anaemia is rare in this country in women of childbearing age, but chronic bleeding from peptic ulceration, aspirin ingestion, or piles may occur. In other countries tapeworms or hookworms may cause a constant chronic blood loss. Treatment is that of the causative condition.

Haemolytic anaemia

Hereditary haemolytic anaemia is also a rare disease in the white population of the United Kingdom, but other races may show a variety of haemolytic anaemias.

Indices of sickle cell anaemia

Blood film
- Red cells
  Polychromasia
  Sickle cells
  Howell-Jolly bodies
- White cells
  Leucocytosis
- Platelets
  Thrombocytosis

Check
- Haemoglobin electrophoresis
- Test partner

Treatment of sickle cell crisis
- Pethidine for pain
- Antibiotic only if accompanying infection
- Oxygen
- Intravenous fluids to maintain hydration
- ? Intravenous bicarbonates for acidaemia
- ? Exchange transfusion

Indices of thalassaemia

Blood film
- Red cells
  ? Polychromasia
  Microcytosis
  Hypochromia
  Sometimes anisocytosis
  Sometimes poikilocytosis
  Target cells present

Haematological values
- Haemoglobin ↓
- Serum iron ↓
- Mean corpuscular volume ↓
- Mean corpuscular haemoglobin ↓

Check
- Haemoglobin electrophoresis
- Test partner

Sickle cell disease

Most adults have haemoglobin A. Defective genes can alter the amino acid sequence of haemoglobin, which may produce symptoms. Haemoglobin S originated in the Middle East but is now found in Africa and the West Indies. Those with haemoglobin C come from West Africa. The partner's blood should be tested and antenatal diagnosis of the fetus is available by direct gene probe from a chorionic villus sample if both partners carry the trait.

In pregnancy a woman with sickle cell disease is at high risk of complications; she deserves special antenatal supervision. Even in experienced hands the perinatal mortality rate can be four times that in a normal population and maternal mortality is also greatly increased. In extreme cases sickling produces crises, leading to sudden pain in the bones, chest, or abdomen after small vessel infarction. A haematological film will show sickle cells and electrophoretic patterns specific to the abnormal haemoglobin. Rates of severe pre-eclampsia are higher, as are the incidences of chest and urinary infections. Intrauterine growth retardation and fetal death occur because of placental infarction.

Higher doses of folate than 5 mg a day have been used to try to reduce the severity of this condition and to prevent the development of any element of folate deficiency anaemia. If a crisis occurs then both haemoglobin concentration and red cell volume should be checked every few hours. Hospital treatment with intravenous hydration, partial exchange transfusion or packed red cell transfusions, and antibiotics may be required. Controversy exists about the value of regular exchange transfusions, but women with haemoglobin concentrations below 6·0 g/dl should have such transfusions before elective delivery. Babies of high risk couples should be tested and followed up if they have sickle cell disease.

Thalassaemia

Most red cells produced by a healthy bone marrow have a life of about 120 days. In thalassaemia the life is much shorter and so anaemia follows because there is a more rapid breakdown than production of cells. Haemoglobin concentration is low but the serum iron concentration is high and the decreased fragility of the red cell can be shown with the sodium chloride test but this is now rarely done.

Again, iron may not be needed if folate concentrations show that stores are adequate but many such women need extra iron as iron deficiency anaemia may accompany thalassaemia. The stress of hypoxia or acidaemia should be avoided as both increase the breakdown rate of red cells.

Women liable to haemoglobinopathies and their antecedents usually come from Mediterranean countries or Asia and are often known to the family doctor beforehand. All such women should have a blood film examined and their blood checked by electrophoresis at the booking clinic. If they are found to be carriers their partner's blood should be checked. If they too are carriers, antenatal diagnosis is available from early chorionic villus sampling and from fetal blood sampling in later pregnancy. Such women are best managed at special combined antenatal-haematological units and should be sent to such hospitals early in pregnancy so that plans can be made to cover all eventualities. If not, as luck would have it, the crisis will always come on Saturday night at 11 30 pm.

Urinary tract infection

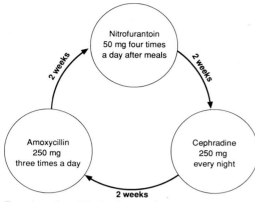

Rotation of antibiotics for persistent bacteriuria.

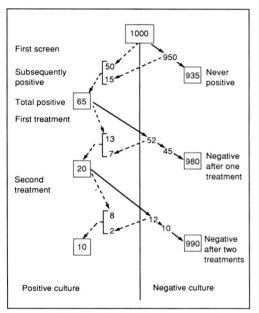

Progress of 1000 women with asymptomatic bacteriuria during pregnancy.

Considerations for pregnancy in chronic renal disease

- Type of disease
  Beware scleroderma, periarteritis nodosa
- Blood pressure
  Diastolic pressure <90 mm Hg
- Renal function
  Plasma creatinine <250 µmol/l
  Plasma urea <10 mmol/l
  No proteinuria
- Review essential drug treatment

Acute urinary infection occurs in about 2% of women during pregnancy. Infection of the urethra and trigone of the bladder is signalled by dysuria and increased frequency of micturition, whereas infection of the upper tract affecting the ureters or kidney produces loin pain and spikes of fever. Often these attacks have occurred before pregnancy, and pregnancy itself is an exacerbating feature.

A midstream urine specimen should be checked for the presence of cells and bacteria (with bacterial sensitivity to antibiotics) before any treatment is started. The woman should drink much more liquid and when her clinical condition warrants it start taking a wide spectrum antibiotic such as ampicillin until the results of the test are known. Antibiotic treatment may have to be changed according to the sensitivity results but usually ampicillin suffices. The woman should rest in bed and drink plenty of liquid (3-4 l a day). Local heat to the loins or suprapubic regions may be helpful; this may sound old fashioned but it is comforting. Alkalination of the urine may be performed, though this is unpleasant and entails taking potassium citrate mixture. It does not help in many cases of urinary tract infection in pregnancy, merely causing the woman to feel more nauseous.

After five days a second midstream urine specimen should be sent to the laboratory. If bacteria are still detected a six week course of three antibiotics in rotation should be prescribed. The three antibiotics may be taken from a list including amoxycillin, nitrofurantoin, and trimethoprin (safe and often used in the second and third trimester).[1]

Asymptomatic bacteriuria

Infection may be low grade and asymptomatic. About 4% of pregnant women have evidence of bacterial infection of the urine; its significance level is arbitrarily set at more than 100 000 bacteria per ml of urine.

If all women are screened early in pregnancy and asymptomatic bacteriuria is detected it is probably wise to treat as the risk of developing acute pyelonephritis in pregnancy is about 30%. Treatment is for five days with an antibiotic to which the bacteria are sensitive. A urine sample should be recultured 14 days later. If bacteria are still present three antibiotics should be prescribed in rotation as mentioned previously.

Any woman with persistent asymptomatic bacteriuria through pregnancy should have her urinary tract checked by intravenous urography after delivery. About 20% of this subgroup will be found to have a structural abnormality of the kidneys, ureters, or bladder.

Chronic renal disease

Most women with chronic renal disease are well known to their general practitioner and have usually been counselled by a renal physician about the risks of pregnancy and the precautions required. In brief, renal function usually improves in pregnancy, and there is no evidence that pregnancy adversely affects the long term prognosis from the renal disease. The outlook in pregnancy is favourable if the patient is not hypertensive and does not have albuminuria before pregnancy. Pregnancy should be carefully supervised by the obstetric and renal team.

Transplant recipients have normal fertility. There is little evidence that the commonly used immunosuppresive agents cause an excess of fetal abnormalities. Episodes of rejection are not more common in pregnancy, but if they occur they usually do so in the puerperium. If the transplanted kidney is in the pelvis a caesarean section may be necessary for mechanical reasons.

I thank Dr John Parker-Williams of St George's Hospital for supplying the blood films and bone marrow aspirate and for advising on the revision of this chapter. The data on iron preparations are taken from the *British National Formulary*. The figure showing screening and treatment of asymptomatic bacteriuria is reproduced by permission of Churchill Livingstone from *Obstetrics* edited by A Turnbull and G Chamberlain.

1 Cunningham FG. Urinary tract infections complicating pregnancy. *Baillieres Clin Obstet Gynaecol* 1987;**1**:891-908.

Recommended reading

de Swiet M. *Medical disorders in obstetric practice.* 2nd ed. Oxford: Blackwell Scientific Publications, 1990.

ABDOMINAL PAIN IN PREGNANCY

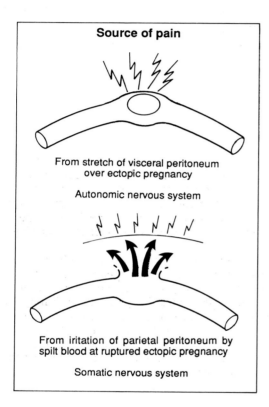

Source of pain

From stretch of visceral peritoneum over ectopic pregnancy

Autonomic nervous system

From iritation of parietal peritoneum by spilt blood at ruptured ectopic pregnancy

Somatic nervous system

Pain in the stomach brings a woman to her doctor's surgery early, especially when she is pregnant. In most such cases the problem is not serious, but all cases need careful assessment as some women will need an immediate opinion at the hospital, some can wait till the next day, and others can wait till the next antenatal clinic. Abdominal pain is diagnosed mostly by clinical means. The history and examination are most important, investigations being less helpful than in other branches of medicine.

The use of ultrasonography by clinical gynaecologists has considerably improved the understanding of pelvic pathology. A vaginal transducer may give better images in early pregnancy than abdominal transducers; however, the laparoscope is still a major investigative tool for lower abdominal pain in early pregnancy. Under appropriate anaesthesia a good view of the pelvis and its organs clinches a diagnosis; in some cases treatment is also possible at the same time.

Pain arises either from inside an organ, involving the covering visceral peritoneum or from later involvement of the parietal peritoneum. The visceral aspects of the pain are poorly localised as they are mediated by the autonomic nervous system. Once the parietal peritoneum is affected, however, impulses travel by the somatic route and localisation may be more specific. Nausea and vomiting occur early in many pelvic conditions as well as in normal pregnancy, which might confuse the picture. Abdominal distension is not usual unless the alimentary tract is involved secondarily; furthermore, it is masked in mid and late pregnancy by the enlarging uterus. Shock may occur if acute pain is accompanied by real hypovolaemia due to blood loss at a ruptured ectopic pregnancy or by relative hypovolaemia after excessive autonomic stimulation from peritoneal irritation of a placental abruption.

For the sake of analysis, in this chapter the commoner causes of abdominal pain in pregnancy are considered as occurring in either late or early pregnancy, even though some conditions can occur in both. The causes will be considered under only one heading, which does not mean, however, that they do not occur in the other half of pregnancy.

Early pregnancy

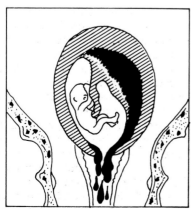

Inevitable miscarriage.

From the uterus

Abortion—One of the commonest causes of pain in early pregnancy is spontaneous miscarriage. The pain usually comes when the miscarriage has passed the threatened stage and is inevitable; the uterus squeezes clot and decidua through the cervical os, thus causing recurrent intermittent pains. The woman may need to be admitted to hospital for evacuation of the uterus. This subject is dealt with in more detail in the chapter on vaginal bleeding in early pregnancy.

Abdominal pain in pregnancy

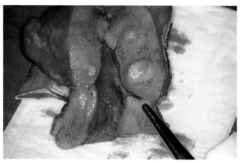

Left: Retroverted uterus (A) and anteverted uterus (B) in early pregnancy.
Right: Management of impacted retroverted uterus during pregnancy (catheterisation).

Retroverted uterus—Retroversion is a common position for a normal uterus. In pregnancy the uterus expands into the abdomen. If adhesions are present, however, this cannot occur; by 10-12 weeks the enlarging uterus fills the pelvis and pain is associated with retention of urine. The urethra is stretched by the uterine bulk and the bladder pushed to the abdomen so that urine cannot pass. These findings can be confirmed by ultrasonography.

Management includes draining the urine with an indwelling catheter. There is little benefit from lying the woman on her front for a few days, although some doctors used to recommend this. The cure eventually comes when the uterus grows into the general abdominal cavity either by moving up entirely or by anterior sacculation, so relieving the urethral stretch.

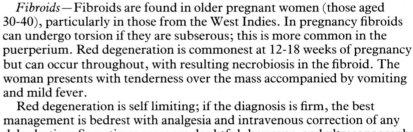

Fibroids are benign quiescent tumours consisting of whorls of fibres and a few cells.

Fibroids—Fibroids are found in older pregnant women (those aged 30-40), particularly in those from the West Indies. In pregnancy fibroids can undergo torsion if they are subserous; this is more common in the puerperium. Red degeneration is commonest at 12-18 weeks of pregnancy but can occur throughout, with resulting necrobiosis in the fibroid. The woman presents with tenderness over the mass accompanied by vomiting and mild fever.

Red degeneration is self limiting; if the diagnosis is firm, the best management is bedrest with analgesia and intravenous correction of any dehydration. Sometimes cases are doubtful, however, and ultrasonography may help to confirm the presence of fibroids, although necrobiosis may not show clearly. In truly doubtful cases, as in a low right sided fibroid that mimicks appendicitis, a laparotomy should be performed to exclude surgically correctable conditions. If red degeneration is diagnosed the surgeon would do well not to remove the fibroid at this stage but to close the abdomen and continue conservative management.

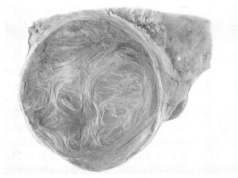

In pregnancy red degeneration may occur suddenly causing severe pain. The fibroid becomes much bigger and softer and is full of red cells. A transverse section looks similar to raw beef.

From the fallopian tube

Ectopic pregnancy—An ectopic pregnancy is one of the most serious conditions that can occur in early pregnancy. Unruptured ectopic pregnancy causes chronic symptoms and needs to be managed in hospital whereas ruptured ectopic pregnancy produces acute symptoms and collapse and needs urgent hospital management. The condition is dealt with in detail in the chapter on vaginal bleeding in early pregnancy.

Torsion—Torsion is uncommon and occurs mainly in younger women during early pregnancy when a long tube may twist on its pedicle accompanied by torsion of the ovary. Torsion is due to the ovary and tube moving from a horizontal to a more vertical position as the uterus enlarges.

The woman has non-specific hypogastric pain and a constant area of tenderness suprapubically on the lateral edge of the rectus abdominis muscle. Ultrasonography does not help but laparoscopy might be useful. A laparotomy is required; if the lateral end of the fallopian tube is non-viable it must be resected; in rare cases the ovary is also ischaemic and requires removal.

> If you do not think of an ectopic pregnancy you will not diagnose one. Always consider unruptured ectopic pregnancy in any young woman at risk who has lower abdominal pain

Abdominal pain in pregnancy

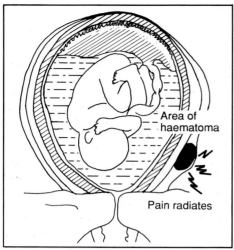

Haematoma of round ligament.

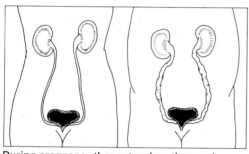

During pregnancy the ureters lengthen and become more tortuous and dilated.

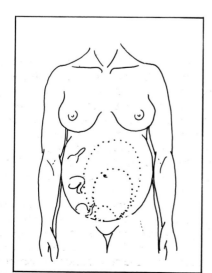

The site of the appendix changes as pregnancy advances.

From the pelvic ligaments

Round ligament—Stretch as the uterus rises in the abdomen pulls on the uterine round ligaments like an inflating hot air balloon tugging its guyropes. Usually the ligaments stretch easily, but if the pull is too rapid small haematomas occur in them. It commonly starts at 16-20 weeks' gestation.

On examination tenderness is localised over the round ligament and often radiates down to the pubic tubercle alongside the symphysis pubis.

Treatment is bed rest, analgesia, and local warmth.

From the ovary

Ovarian tumours—In early pregnancy an ovarian cystic tumour may rupture to release the contents of the cyst, which irritate the parietal peritoneum. Alternatively, bleeding may occur into a corpus luteal cyst, producing sudden pain localised poorly to one side of the abdomen with tenderness detectable on that side. An ultrasound scan may confirm the diagnosis, and a laparotomy is usually required to remove only the part of the ovary containing the cyst. It used to be considered that a corpus luteum, the main site of progesterone manufacture in the first 12 weeks of pregnancy, could not be removed without the woman aborting. This is no longer considered immutable. The trophoblast that is to become the placenta is already making progesterone; such problems do not usually occur until after the eighth week of pregnancy. If the obstetrician is concerned he or she could prescribe exogenous progestogens of the non-virilising type, but their use is unproved.

Torsion of an ovarian tumour is less common in pregnancy, but a dermoid may undergo twisting, producing colicky pain. A tender mass may sometimes be palpated, either abdominally or bimanually, and the treatment consists of removal of the tumour at laparotomy. This is safest between 14 and 24 weeks of gestation.

Extrapelvic causes

Vomiting—Though many women who vomit in pregnancy have little upset, vomiting may be sufficiently severe to cause muscle ache from stretch. The upper abdominal wall is tender and no specific masses can be felt. If a woman is vomiting this much it is probably wise to admit her to hospital for intravenous fluids, antiemetic treatment, and sedation to allow her intestinal tract some peace. The pain usually settles down as the vomiting decreases.

Pyelonephritis—Stasis in the urinary tract associated with ascending urinary infection often follows dilatation of the ureters (due to raised progesterone concentrations) and the pressure of the increasing uterus on the bladder. It is most likely in mid-pregnancy, when the woman presents with vomiting, symptoms of fever, and low hypogastric or loin pain. She will be feverish and have ill defined tenderness over the suprapubic region and fairly precise tenderness in one or other subcostal angle. A midstream urine specimen may contain pus cells and bacteria.

Until the results of urine analysis are known the woman should have bed rest and be treated with local heat, a high fluid diet, analgesics, and broad spectrum antibiotics. The result of the urine test may indicate another antibiotic but often the patient's condition has improved by this time. Most women with pyelonephritis should be treated in hospital as intravenous fluid and antibiotics may be needed and uterine activity may be stimulated by the accompanying fever. Recurrent or resistant urinary infection in pregnancy deserves follow up after the baby is born. A high proportion of such women have a structural abnormality of the urinary tract.

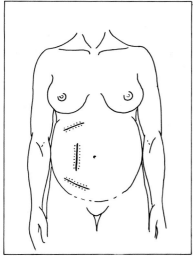

The site of incision for appendicectomy during pregnancy. This rises with increasing uterine size and is shown at 12, 24, and 36 weeks of gestation above.

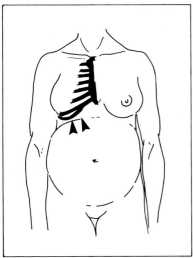

Pain in cholecystitis.

Appendicitis—Appendicitis and pregnancy both occur in young women and therefore may occur concurrently by chance. The incidence of appendicitis in pregnancy is not increased but its diagnosis may be more difficult. For this reason and because of a reluctance to operate appendicitis used to have a high mortality and morbidity in pregnancy.

As it grows the uterus displaces the caecum from the right iliac fossa upwards and sideways, so the inflamed appendix may present with symptoms and signs in unexpected places. No longer tucked into the right iliac fossa, the appendix is now in the general abdomen and is less easy to wall off by omentum and gut when it becomes inflamed; generalised peritonitis is commoner in pregnant than non-pregnant women.

A history may elicit the characteristic pain shift, although it might not be localised to the right iliac fossa. Nausea and anorexia occur, sometimes confused by the symptoms of pregnancy. The tenderness over the appendix will shift higher as pregnancy continues. The treatment is operation, the incision being placed over the point of maximum tenderness marked by the surgeon before anaesthesia. Occasionally the results of a rectal examination can be falsely reassuring if the appendix has migrated from the area reached by an examining finger.

The previous reluctance to operate must be overcome; anyone suspected of having appendicitis in pregnancy should have a laparotomy by an experienced obstetric surgeon. Even in late pregnancy, caesarean section is not necessary at the same time unless the woman is in labour; women can have normal vaginal deliveries within a few days of an appendicectomy.

Other causes—Cholecystitis is commoner among women who live in or originate from countries whose residents characteristically have high cholesterol diets such as Australia and New Zealand. The pain is usually upper abdominal with tenderness centred on the eighth or ninth rib tip. Treatment in the absence of jaundice is drainage or removal, depending on the surgical need.

Volvulus of large bowel can occur in pregnancy, though it presents more characteristically in the puerperium.

Small bowel colic may follow an attack of gasteroentritis. Urinary lithiasis occurs in the same frequency in pregnancy as in non-pregnant women pregnancy in areas of the country where the prevalence is increased.

Late pregnancy

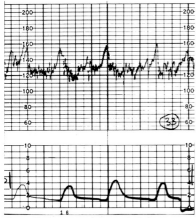

A cardiotocograph in early labour showing the fetal heart rate above the regular uterine contractions every three minutes.

From the uterus

Uterine contractions—All pregnancies end in labour, which can occur well before 40 weeks of gestation. Premature labour can present with abdominal pain, taking the woman and sometimes her general practitioner by surprise. Usually the pain is intermittent and recurrent and the uterus can be felt contracting coincidentally with the pain. There may be a loss of mucus or a little blood from the vagina, and on vaginal examination the cervix is soft, thin, taken up, and sometimes dilated. When labour is very preterm (26-32 weeks) the woman should perhaps be transferred to a hospital with a good neonatal unit rather than necessarily to the one where she has booked (see the chapter on preterm labour).

Placental abruption—Separation of the placenta from its bed before the third stage of labour is painful and results in shock (see chapter on vaginal bleeding in early pregnancy). The pain is produced by blood tearing into the myometrium, separating the fibres widely, and finally reaching the visceral peritoneum. This also produces a tonic uterine contraction. Treatment is immediate delivery probably by caesarean section if the baby is still alive and otherwise vaginally promptly.

Abdominal pain in pregnancy

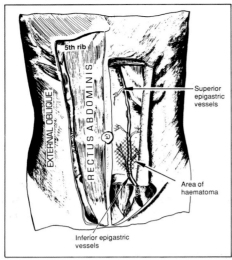

A rectus haematoma usually arises from the inferior epigastric vessels deep in the rectus muscle.

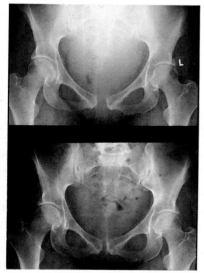

Above: Pelvis immediately after delivery showing dehiscence of pubic symphysis. Below: Same pelvis six weeks later. Imaging by ultrasonography reduces the risks of irradiation in a young woman.

Extraperitoneal causes

Pregnancy induced hypertension—In severe fulminating pregnancy induced hypertension a woman may complain of hypogastric pain associated with vomiting. She will probably have raised blood pressure and proteinuria with oedema and be known to be hypertensive. There may also be visual signs (outlined in the chapter on raised blood pressure in pregnancy). The pain is due to stretch of the peritoneum over the liver after the organ has become oedematous. Treatment of the pregnancy induced hypertension will resolve symptoms.

Rectus haematoma—Very rarely the rectus muscle may dehisce or the inferior epigastric veins behind the muscle rupture. As the anterior abdominal wall is greatly overstretched by the uterus, a fit of sneezing could cause this. Pain is severe and usually localised to one segment of the muscle. Blood loss is slight with the haematoma but increases if the veins rupture; investigations are not much help. Rectus haematoma is diagnosed from the fact that pain and tenderness worsen when the woman contracts the rectus muscles by raising her head. Ultrasonography is helpful.

If the diagnosis is firm management is conservative, but in doubtful cases a laparotomy should be performed, and haematoma behind the rectus muscle confirms the diagnosis.

Pelvic arthropathy—Relaxation of the ligaments guarding the pelvic joints follows the secretion of the hormone relaxin. This allows appreciable separation of the symphysis pubis, giving abdominal pain that is much aggravated by walking. In extreme cases weight bearing is impossible and the woman has to retire to bed completely. Treatment is rest; binders are of little help. It may take up to two months to resolve after delivery, but it usually does slowly get better. Severe cases may last for up to a year, and long term follow up is wise.

Conclusions

> Early abdominal examination will often help differentiate serious from non-serious conditions

Most women who present with abdominal pain in pregnancy may have nothing serious the matter. Pain can, however, lead the doctor to diagnose a serious condition, when action needs to be taken. As investigations play a small part in many of these diagnoses, experienced general practitioners can often diagnose its cause and continue the management of many women at home, but if there is any doubt the local obstetric department ought to be consulted.

Recommended reading

Burdenell JM, Wile PL. *Medical and surgical problems in pregnancy.* Bristol: John Wright, 1984.

RAISED BLOOD PRESSURE IN PREGNANCY

Some accepted definitions of raised blood pressure

Hypertension
- Mild—diastolic blood pressure >90 mm Hg
- Severe—diastolic blood pressure > 110 mm Hg

Pregnancy induced hypertension
- Mild—diastolic blood pressure >90 mm Hg after the 20th week of pregnancy with no raised blood pressure beforehand and no proteinuria
- Moderate—diastolic blood pressure >100 mm Hg after the 20th week of pregnancy with no raised blood pressure beforehand and no proteinuria
- Severe—diastolic blood pressure >90 mm Hg after the 20th week of pregnancy with no raised blood pressure beforehand but with any degree of proteinuria

One of the original aims of promaternity (antenatal) care in 1901 was the prevention of fits and convulsions due to eclampsia, which was often associated with pre-eclampsia. The term pre-eclampsia has been replaced in later years as eclampsia now occurs rarely.

Raised blood pressure affects the fetus as well as the mother. In the later weeks of pregnancy it may fall into one of several categories.
- Chronic hypertension is present before the 20th week and has causes outside pregnancy
- Pregnancy induced hypertension develops after the 20th week of pregnancy and usually resolves within 10 days after delivery
- Pregnancy induced hypertension with proteinuria used to be called pre-eclampsia and occurs mostly in primigravidas
- Pregnancy induced hypertension with or without proteinuria may be superimposed on chronic hypertension and this is a most dangerous combination, the effects of pregnancy being added to those of chronic hypertension
- Eclampsia is a convulsive condition usually associated with proteinuric hypertension.

Causes

The cause of pregnancy induced hypertension is now almost completely understood, with reasonable educated guesses being possible in unknown cases. The primary defect is failure of the second wave of trophoblastic invasion into the decidua. Usually the trophoblast invades the entire length of the spiral arteries by 22 weeks of gestation. This leads to an appreciable fall in peripheral resistance and therefore a fall in blood pressure. In addition, as the trophoblast usually removes all the muscle coat of the spiral arteries, blood flows unimpeded into the intervillous space, gushing like a fountain over the villous tree that contains the fetal vessels. This ensures adequate time for exchange of oxygen, nutrients, and the waste products of metabolism.

Permutations of hypertensive disease in pregnant and non-pregnant women.

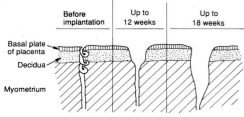

The invasion of spiral arteries by the trophoblast converts them into deltas and so improves blood flow.

If the second wave of trophoblastic invasion fails the peripheral resistance does not fall and the haemodynamic mechanisms are not reset for the increased vascular space of pregnancy. Furthermore, the muscle coats retained by the spiral arterioles are sensitive to circulating pressor agents, particularly angiotensin II. At the spiral arterioles the reduced volume of trophoblast leads to an imbalance in the prostacyclin-thromboxane system. The comparative overproduction of thromboxane encourages vasospasm of the spiral arteries and also local platelet aggregation. The lower concentrations of prostacyclin remove the protection that pregnancy offers against angiotensin II.

Raised blood pressure in pregnancy

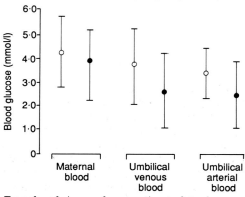

Transfer of glucose from mother to fetus in babies who show normal growth (○) and in those who are small for gestational age (●).

The damaged muscle coating and intima of the spiral arteries undergoes acute atherosis, an accelerated form of arteriosclerosis that further narrows and then occludes the arterioles. A further increase in blood pressure follows, and the decrease in perfusion of the intervillous space leads commonly to intrauterine growth retardation.

Low dose aspirin may abolish pregnancy induced hypertension in patients at risk and moderates the disease once established. The mode of action is irreversible poisoning of platelet cyclo-oxygenase. This probably prevents or delays clotting in the spiral arterioles.

The effects of pregnancy induced hypertension on organs other than the placenta are mediated by the hypertension or by activation of the complement system. This causes immune complexes to be deposited on the basement membrane of the kidney and allows protein to leak into the urine. In severe disease platelets are both consumed and activated so that coagulopathy may follow.

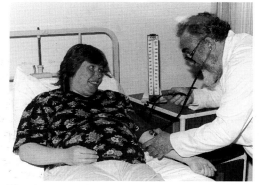

Blood pressure measurement is a simple and useful screening test when performed repeatedly by standardised techniques. All doctors and midwives in a unit should use the same criterion for diastolic pressure—probably phase IV Korotkoff sound.

Management

Though pregnancy induced hypertension develops out of the blue, particularly in first pregnancies, many women who already have hypertension will wonder about becoming pregnant and the effects that the pregnancy may have on their underlying hypertension. This matter should be considered carefully before a woman becomes pregnant, and if necessary the woman should be referred to a local prepregnancy advisory service.

Generally speaking, if the blood pressure is not very high, or it can be kept low with antihypertensive drugs, and if there is no concomitant proteinuria before pregnancy most women will have a successful pregnancy but will need to be admitted to hospital. They should continue their antihypertensive treatment in pregnancy.

Women with renal damage already leading to proteinuria and those who have diastolic pressures above 100 mm Hg despite adequate antihypertensive treatment should be investigated more thoroughly. Such women have a three to seven times increased risk above background that they will develop pregnancy induced hypertension on top of their disease and the prognosis is worse for both mother and baby.

The ideal start to the management of pregnancy induced hypertension, with or without proteinuria, is to detect it early. Each visit to the antenatal clinic includes a blood pressure recording. Recently, women likely to develop pregnancy induced hypertension have been detected before this happens at 24 weeks by the use of Doppler measurements of blood flow velocity in the placental bed, from which a measure of placental vascular resistance is derived.[1] Doppler investigation may become available as a screening test in the next few years, providing, for example, an indicator of which women would benefit from low dose aspirin.

Once raised blood pressure is established bed rest is usually central to primary management. Without accompanying proteinuria, the woman may be treated at home, where bed rest must take priority over everything else, including work at home or outside and care of other members of the family. If the hypertension increases despite proper bed rest, or proteinuria follows, admission to hospital is required.

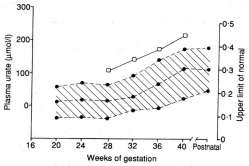

Changes in plasma urate concentration from 16 weeks of gestation showing 10th, 50th, and 90th centiles and the accepted upper limit of normal values (□——□).

In hospital bed rest will be reinforced and the condition will be monitored by using ultrasound measurements of the growth of the fetus, Doppler measurements of blood velocity in both placental bed and umbilical arteries, and cardiotocographic measurements of variations in the fetal heart rate. Plasma urate concentrations are the only useful biochemical indicator of deterioration, and a fall in the platelet count reflects severe disease. The management of severe hypertension now no longer includes treatment with sedatives or diuretics; sedatives tend merely to reduce the mother's level of consciousness and cross the placenta, causing depression of the fetal central and peripheral nervous systems. Similarly, diuretics are of little use, except for the relief of acutely painful oedema. They may even be harmful by reducing plasma volume and therefore perfusion of the placental bed.

Drugs and dosages used in treatment of pregnancy induced hypertension

Drug	Route	Dosage	Comment
Centrally acting drugs			
Clonidine	Oral	500-100 µg three times a day	
Methyldopa	Oral	250-1000 mg daily	Safe to use for many years
Vasodilators			
Sodium nitroprusside	Intravenous	0·3-1·0 µg/kg/min	Potentially toxic to fetus
Hydralazine	Oral	25-50 twice a day	
	Intravenous	5-20 mg over 20 minutes	Drug of choice to give intravenously in emergency hypertension
β Adrenoceptor blockers			
Atenolol	Intravenous	2·5 mg at 1 mg/min	
	Oral	50-100 mg daily	
Propanolol	Oral	80-160 mg daily	May reduce placental perfusion
α and β Adrenoceptor blockers			
Labetalol	Intravenous	50 mg over a minute	Water soluble and so crosses placenta; may not be effective in acute problem
	Oral	100-200 mg daily	

Antihypertensive drugs are useful in protecting the mother's circulation, mostly against the risk of a stroke. They have no effect on the progression of the pregnancy induced hypertension or on fetal growth but they help to maintain the pregnancy longer to allow the fetus to become more mature. These drugs tend to be kept for women whose hypertension increases despite bed rest; treatment should be started only in women who are inpatients. Methyldopa is still the commonest oral drug used for a few weeks. Hydralazine is given intravenously as first aid in acutely deteriorating hypertension. Some β blockers, such as atenolol, or combined α and β blockers, such as labetalol, are gaining in popularity because of their better control.

> The ultimate treatment of pregnancy induced hypertension is delivery

The final and ultimate treatment of pregnancy induced hypertension is delivery. Induction of labour or caesarean section should be reserved until the fetus is mature enough for the neonatal facilities available, but it must be used when the condition deteriorates. Two changes in managing pregnancy induced hypertension in this decade have considerably altered the outlook for mother and fetus. Firstly, use of antihypertensive drugs to allow the fetus to spend longer in the uterus has spread rapidly and widely from its epicentre in Oxford.[2] Formerly, such drugs were thought to affect the fetus deleteriously and so their use in pregnancy was restricted. Now most obstetricians use them, and by reducing maternal risk pregnancy is prolonged by a few more weeks so that the child is more mature. Secondly, the obstetrician's reluctance to perform a caesarean section earlier in pregnancy has diminished. With improved intensive neonatal care, caesarean section as early as 26 weeks gives a reasonable chance of fetal survival. The worst effects of prolonged renal and cerebral damage are reduced for the mother and the fetus is delivered before being affected by serious chronic hypoxia in utero.

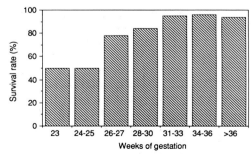

Survival to discharge by gestational age at a typical neonatal intensive care unit in 1989.

The treatment of women with severe pregnancy induced hypertension is best performed in special regional hypertension units, where neonatal and obstetrical care is planned together. The Confidential Enquiries into Maternal Deaths have shown for years that each regional health authority should have one or more such designated units. A woman with or at risk of severe pregnancy induced hypertension should be admitted to such a unit to obtain the best concentrated and coordinated obstetric and neonatal care.

The future management of pregnancy induced hypertension may lie in the reduction of platelet agglutination during early pregnancy, so preventing damage of the placental bed. This might halt the whole cascade of problems. Aspirin in early pregnancy would block the cyclo-oxygenase enzymes of the platelets so that they would not be able to produce thromboxane. Recent studies have shown that low dose aspirin (75 mg a day) may be helpful in mitigating the worst effects of pregnancy induced hypertension with proteinuria.[3]

Raised blood pressure in pregnancy
Eclampsia

Imminent eclampsia

The old term fulminating pre-eclampsia is less often used, but semantics are not as important as the recognition of this severe, acute change in a woman's condition. Having had moderate or even severe but symptom free pregnancy induced hypertension with proteinuria, the woman suddenly starts to produce symptoms. She may have frontal headaches and visual symptoms with jagged, angular flashes at the periphery of her visual fields and loss of vision in areas, both symptoms being due to cerebral oedema. She often has epigastric pain due to stretch of the peritoneum over the oedematous liver. In addition, some women have a curious itch confined to the mask region of the face. On examination her blood pressure may be much raised above previous readings or proteinuria may increase sharply; she may have increased and brisk reflex reponses at knee and clonus. This woman needs urgent hypotensive and anticonvulsant treatment. If she is at home she should be admitted under the cover of a flying squad, with intravenous diazepam and, if necessary, hydralazine running continuously. Diazepam prevents fits and hydralazine reduces blood pressure.

Eclampsia

Convulsions associated with pregnancy induced hypertension are termed eclampsia; they are very similar in form to those of epilepsy. Occasionally women in the beginning of the third trimester have eclamptic fits, having had perfectly normal blood pressure readings and urine test results within the previous few weeks at the routine visits to the antenatal clinic. Most women with eclampsia, however, give prodromal signs of pregnancy induced hypertension with proteinuria in pregnancy; the fits may develop in labour or the puerperium, the first day after birth having the highest risk.

The general practitioner's first move is to control the fits and prevent them causing damage to the woman. She should be laid on her side and an airway established. Intravenous diazepam is given to stop the fits, usually about 20-40 mg; this is followed by intramuscular injections (10 mg) or a continuous intravenous infusion. Recently, phenytoin has been used to prevent the recurrence of fits.

In Great Britain doctors are reluctant to use magnesium sulphate, which is widely used in America and is an excellent anticonvulsant. Should the blood pressure be steeply raised, intravenous hydralazine is the best treatment either in a 5 mg bolus at 20 minutes or given intravenously as 25 mg in 500 ml of Hartmann's solution, with the drip rate titrated against the woman's blood pressure. This is best administered through a separate drip set so that anticonvulsant and antihypertension treatments can be given at different rates according to clinical needs. If the woman is in labour or induction is considered an epidural anaesthetic may be helpful, both to lower the blood pressure and to reduce the tendency to fit by removing the pain of intrauterine contractions. Any tendency of the women to have increased blood clotting should be excluded.

The ultimate treatment of eclampsia is delivery. Should eclampsia occur at home the woman must be transported to hospital by a flying squad immediately. Although rare, eclampsia still occurs in this country and in the triennium 1985-7 caused 12 maternal deaths in England and Wales.

Delivery of the infant

It must be emphasised that the ultimate cure of pregnancy induced hypertension and eclampsia is delivery. The obstetrician must weigh the answers to two often conflicting questions:

- When would it be safer for the mother to be delivered?

- When would it be safer for the baby to be outside the uterus rather than on the wrong side of a failing placental exchange system?

Maternal considerations may be judged by the speed of deterioration of the condition (blood pressure and proteinuria) and the expected proximity of severe complications such as eclampsia. Fetal state is best assessed by measuring the circulation supplying the fetus both in the spiral arteries

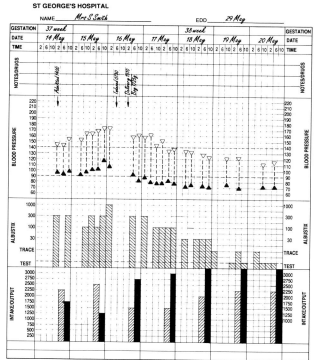

Blood pressure chart of a woman with severe pregnancy induced hypertension before and after delivery.

coming to the placental bed and in the umbilical vessels; if there is time serial ultrasound measurements of fetal growth are useful. If these data are available a rational decision can be made about the timing of the removal of the fetus from the hostile environment in a centre with a neonatal intensive care unit. Women should be transferred early to regional centres for hypertension in pregnancy when it is obvious that the pregnancy induced hypertension is not going to settle with bed rest and mild or moderate drug treatments. If a regional health authority has no regional centre it should find and fund one now as many difficult problems arising from hypertension in pregnancy need expert care and the use of special investigations and management. There is little place for heroic management in peripheral hospitals with a greatly compromised baby and mother afterward.

Mode of delivery after control of eclampsia

Factors favouring vaginal delivery

- Multiparous mother
- Stable blood pressure and cerebral irritability
- Ripe cervix
- Mature fetus (>1500 g estimated weight)
- Cephalic presentation
- Normally grown fetus
- Fetus in good state to stand uterine contractions

Factors favouring caesarean section

- Primiparous mother
- Unstable blood pressure control or cerebral irritability
- Unripe cervix
- Immature fetus (<1500 g estimated weight)
- Breech presentation
- Intrauterine growth retardation
- Poor prognosis of fetal state from Doppler blood flow rates or cardiotocography

Conclusions

Early diagnosis can modify some of the effects of pregnancy induced hypertension

Once it has been decided that it would be safer for the mother and the baby that delivery should occur the method and route of that delivery should be considered. If it is thought unsafe for the baby to undergo the contractions of labour, or if the baby is immature or has an inappropriate presentation, a caesarean section is indicated. If the mother's condition is deteriorating rapidly, again, the abdominal route would be swifter. If, however, the woman has a ripe cervix, the hypertensive state is not worsening rapidly, and the fetus is in an acceptable position and of reasonable maturity induction of labour should be performed with prostaglandin pessaries or membrane rupture, depending on the usage in the labour ward. An unripe cervix and a need for speedy delivery would also be grounds for a caesarean section.

Intrauterine growth retardation is associated with pregnancy induced hypertension. The two go together and share common causes. Narrowing of the placental bed vessels reduces nutrition to the fetus in pregnancy just as it reduces available oxygen during labour. Many fetuses born to women with unmanaged pregnancy induced hypertension are small for their gestational age. Unfortunately so are many fetuses born to women who are very well managed; the fetal growth retardation therefore probably starts long before conventional management of the mother starts.

Pregnancy induced hypertension is still a major problem in antenatal medicine but many of its worst effects can be mitigated by early diagnosis from blood pressure readings at clinic visits. The future includes predictive Doppler measurements of blood flow and preventive treatment, which may include aspirin. If the condition is severe the mother's and baby's prognoses will be greatly improved if a regional hypertension in pregnancy unit is used.

1 Steel SA, Pearce JM, McParland P, Chamberlain GVP. Doppler ultrasound as a screening test of severe pre-eclampsia. *Lancet* 1990;335:1548-51.
2 Redman CWG, Beilin LJ, Bonnar J. Treatment of hypertension in pregnancy with methyldopa: blood pressure control and side effects. *Br J Obstet Gynaecol* 1977;84:419-26.
3 McParland P, Pearce JM, Chamberlain GVP. Doppler ultrasound and aspirin in the recognition and prevention of pregnancy induced hypertension. *Lancet* 1990;355:1552-6.

Recommended reading

Redman CWG. Hypertension in pregnancy. In: Turnbull A, Chamberlain G, eds. *Obstetrics*. London: Churchill Livingstone, 1989: 515-42.

The figure showing transfer of glucose is reproduced by permission of Blackwell Scientific Publications from *Modern Antenatal Care of the Fetus* edited by G Chamberlain and that showing change in plasma urate concentrations by permission of Churchill Livingstone from *Obstetrics* edited by A Turnbull and G Chamberlain.

ANTEPARTUM HAEMORRHAGE

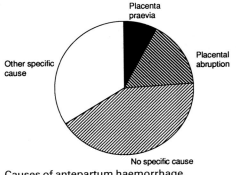

Causes of antepartum haemorrhage.

Antepartum haemorrhage is bleeding from the genital tract between 28 completed weeks of pregnancy and the onset of labour. Many of the causes exist before this time and can produce bleeding. Although strictly speaking such bleeding is not an antepartum haemorrhage, the old fashioned definition is not appropriate for modern neonatal management.

The placental bed is the commonest site of antepartum haemorrhage; in a few cases bleeding is from local causes in the genital tract whereas in a substantial remainder the bleeding has no obvious cause but it is probably still from the placental bed.

Placental abruption

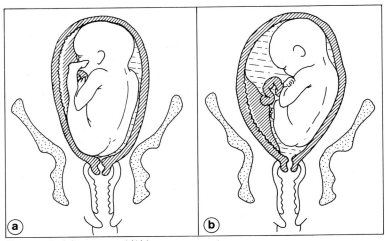

Placenta in (a) upper and (b) lower segment.

If the placenta separates before delivery the denuded placental bed bleeds. If the placenta is implanted in the upper segment of the uterus the bleeding is termed an abruption; if a part of the placenta is in the lower uterine segment it is designated a placenta praevia.

Placental abruption may entail only a small area of placental separation. The clot remains between placenta and placental bed but little or no blood escapes through the cervix (concealed abruption). Further separation causes further loss of blood, which oozes between the membranes and decidua, passing down through the cervix to appear at the vulva (revealed abruption).

In addition, the vessels around the side of the placenta may tear (marginal vein bleeding), which is clinically indistinguishable from placental abruption. The differentiation between revealed and concealed abruption is not very useful. The important factor is the amount of placenta separated from its bed and the coincident spasm of the placental bed vessels. If exchange is reduced enough it will lead to fetal death.

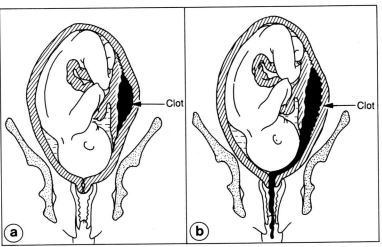

(a) Concealed and (b) revealed placental abruption.

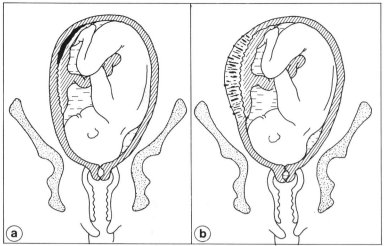

The degree of fetal affect depends on the amount of separation and spasm of placental bed vessels (*a*), while the maternal affect depends on the amount of tissue damage to the myometrium (*b*).

Pathology

Bleeding between the placenta and its bed causes separation; as more blood is forced between the layers detachment becomes wider. Blood also tracks between the myometrial fibres, sometimes reaching the peritoneal surface. The mother's pain and shock depend on the amount of tissue damage rather than on the volume of bleeding. The fetal state depends on both the amount of separation and the spasm of the blood vessels in the placental bed.

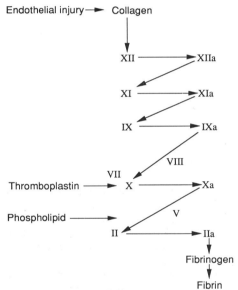

Points in the clotting cascade at which the sequelae of a placental abruption can intervene and so lead to disseminated intravascular coagulopathy.

Sometimes amniotic fluid or trophoblast tissue is forced into the maternal circulation after a placental abruption. Thromboplastins start disseminated intravascular coagulation, which in a mild case is coped with by the maternal fibrinolytic system, but if the amniotic fluid embolus is large maternal plasma fibrinogen concentration is depleted. Uterine bleeding continues with activation of the maternal fibrinolytic system; widespread deprivation of fibrin and fibrinogen follows, producing a vicious circle of more bleeding.

The cause of placental abruption is unknown. It happens more commonly in association with a uterine abnormality and there is a 10% risk or recurrence if it has occurred previously. Conditions of uterine overstretch such as polyhydramnios and twin pregnancy are associated with abruption if amniotic fluid is released suddenly at the induction of labour.

Diagnosis

The woman presents with poorly localised abdominal pain over the uterus; there may be some dark red vaginal bleeding or clots. Depending on the degree of placental separation and uterine spasm, clinical shock may also be present. If the abruption is severe the uterus contracts tonically so that fetal parts cannot be felt; the fetus may be dead with no fetal heart detectable. Ultrasonography may show the retroplacental clot but gives no measure of the extent of functional disorder.

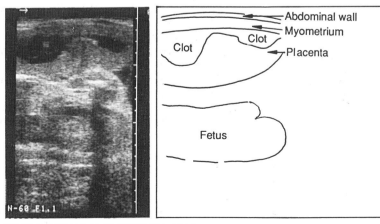

Ultrasound scan of placental abruption.

The differential diagnosis is from:

● Placenta praevia, which is not usually accompanied by pain, often results in brighter bleeding as the blood is fresher and rarely results in much shock

● Rupture of the uterus, which may present with a similar picture to placental abruption

● Red degeneration of a uterine fibroid at 24-30 weeks' gestation

● Bleeding from a ruptured vessel on the surface of the pregnant uterus, which is rare.

The diagnosis of abruption is finally confirmed after delivery by finding organised clot firmly adherent to the placenta.

Management

A woman with an abruption has a potentially dangerous condition that requires all the facilities the general practitioner can get. She must be admitted to hospital quickly, if necessary with the help of a flying squad. Group O rhesus negative blood may be required urgently in the home and, if not, supportive intravenous treatment should be established. Hartmann's solution or saline may be used at first followed by a plasma expander. The general practitioner should take blood samples first for crossmatching. Pain may be relieved by morphine, and the woman must be transferred to hospital when her condition is stable. In a very mild case the flying squad may not be needed but the woman should be escorted by her general practitioner to hospital.

In hospital the anti-shock measures will be continued and blood given. At least four units of blood must be crossmatched, irrespective of the scant external blood loss; fresh frozen plasma and platelets should be available. Central venous pressures are a guide to the amount of blood required. Once the condition is stabilising delivery should take place immediately by caesarean section. This can be a difficult operation needing a senior obstetrician. If the fetus is dead, artificial rupture of the membranes usually leads to a rapid labour.

After a mild abruption and if the fetus is immature and lives the woman may continue the pregnancy under controlled conditions. She will stay in hospital with antenatal monitoring until the fetus is mature enough for delivery. In cases occurring very early in gestation the woman may have to be transferred for delivery to a regional unit with intensive neonatal facilities available.

Severe abruption may lead to severely disordered blood clotting which must be managed with the help of a haematologist. After delivery fluid balance should be carefully managed and urine output must be recorded hourly. Oliguria, not due to reduced plasma volume, is usually the result of acute tubular necrosis, though in rare cases acute cortical necrosis may occur. The help of anaesthetists trained in intensive care and of a renal physician will be needed.

Management of placental abruption

- Get the woman to hospital urgently
- Replace real correct volume of blood lost
- Monitor central venous pressure
- If fetus alive and mature:
    Caesarean section
    Check for disseminated intravascular
        coagulopathy
    Check renal function and urinary output
- If fetus dead:
    Induce (artificial rupture of the
        membranes)

Placenta praevia

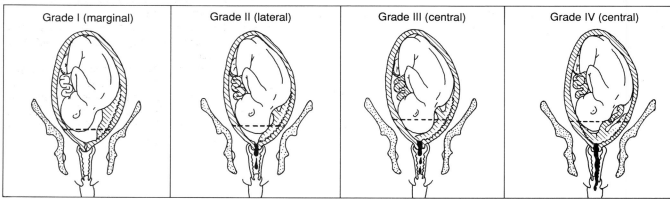

The older grades of placenta praevia were 1-4. More recently they are described as marginal, lateral, and central.

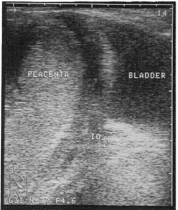

Ultrasound scan of placenta praevia.

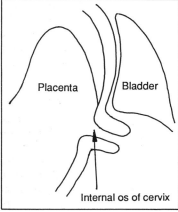

The blastocyst usually implants in the thicker, receptive endometrium of the upper uterus, but occasionally it implants in the endometrium of the isthmus or over a previous lower segment uterine scar. Then invasion by the trophoblast secures the embryo and when the uterus grows to form a lower segment later in pregnancy some part of the placenta is implanted there.

About a tenth of all antepartum haemorrhages are due to placenta praevia, the proportion increasing with more thorough investigative ultrasonography. In the last weeks of pregnancy the lower segment stretches whereas the placenta is comparatively inelastic. In consequence, the placenta is peeled off the uterine wall with bleeding from the placental bed. A placenta praevia may be detected by ultrasonography in the mid-trimester but usually little bleeding occurs until the lower segment is formed.

Diagnosis

A woman with placenta praevia may have bright red, painless bleeding. It comes unexpectedly, blood often being found on waking in the morning. The woman is in no way shocked and may want to ignore the symptom as she feels normal.

A few women present with a persistent transverse lie or breech presentation in late pregnancy. The possibility of placenta praevia should always be considered in such a case and an ultrasound scan requested urgently. The result may lead to the woman's admission to hospital, although she has had no bleeding.

In a third group of women a placenta praevia is diagnosed incidentally on ultrasound examination. This finding is common in the middle weeks of pregnancy. A low lying placenta diagnosed at 18 weeks' gestation is often normally sited by 32 weeks. About 5% of women present with a low lying placenta at 18 weeks but only 1% of them have a placenta praevia at delivery. The upper segment of the uterus grows and the placental site moves with it as the lower segment is formed. If not, such women should be treated in the same way as others diagnosed clinically because the risk of bleeding in late pregnancy is as great.

The uterine spasm of placental abruption does not occur in placenta praevia and the fetus can be easily felt. It is usually alive with good heart tones. The woman's degree of shock will vary directly with the amount of blood lost. If shock is moderate the woman needs admission to hospital with the help of a flying squad and the blood that it carries. If blood loss is slight she can go to the hospital more conventionally but she needs to be warned of the probable diagnosis.

No vaginal examinations should be performed on any woman who bleeds in late pregnancy until a placenta praevia has been excluded by ultrasonography. If this principle is broached, further separation of the placenta may occur with very heavy, and sometimes fatal, haemorrhage. Any woman who presents to a general practitioner with vaginal bleeding in late pregnancy should be considered to have a placenta praevia until the diagnosis is disproved. She must be referred to a hospital for an urgent appointment that day. If necessary, she should be admitted if ultrasound investigations cannot be performed straight away.

In hospital blood is crossmatched and the placental site demonstrated by ultrasonography. The older diagnostic radioisotope studies and soft tissue *x* ray examinations now have no place.

Once placenta praevia is diagnosed, the aim of treatment is to maintain the pregnancy until the fetus is mature enough to be delivered; at 36-38 weeks an elective caesarean section will be performed unless the placenta praevia is a minor one with the fetal presenting part below it. Should the placenta be anterior, the operation may be difficult with much blood loss and should be performed by a senior obstetrician.

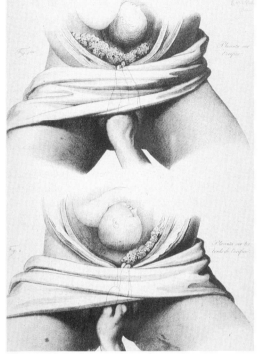

These old steel engravings show what a vaginal examination could do to a placenta praevia (central (above) and lateral (below)). NEVER DO A VAGINAL EXAMINATION UNLESS PLACENTA PRAEVIA IS EXCLUDED.

Other specific causes of bleeding

General

Few haemorrhagic diseases occur in young women but vaginal bleeding may occur in von Willebrand's disease, Hodgkin's disease, and leukaemia. All are probably known about beforehand, and the diagnosis is confirmed from the results of haematological studies.

Local

Lesions of the cervix and vagina cause slight bleeding, often only a smear of blood and mucus. Moderate bleeding may occur with a carcinoma of the cervix—rare in women of childbearing age—or varicose veins of the vulva and lower vagina. Lesser bleeding is more likely from a polyp or an erosion of the cervix. Monilia infection may be accompanied by spotting as plaques of fungoid tissue are separated from the vaginal walls.

Causes of antepartum haemorrhage from the lower genital tract

Cause	Characteristic bleeding
Cervical ectropion	Smear of blood loss often with mucous loss
Cervical polyp	Spotting of blood
Cervical cancer	Smear of blood on touch (rare, but diagnosis is important) May bleed heavily
Vaginal moniliasis	Spotting of blood with white or pink discharge
Vaginal varicose veins	Occasionally heavy bleeding

Antepartum haemorrhage

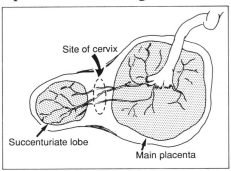

Vasa praevia. A succenturiate lobe is separated from the main body of the placenta. Should the vessels run over the cervix, when the cervix dilates they may be torn so that fetal blood is lost.

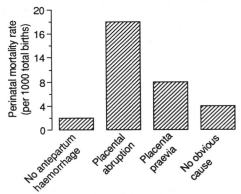

The relative risks of increased perinatal mortality from antepartum haemorrhage compared with those in pregnancies with no such haemorrhage.

All these causes can be diagnosed readily by using a speculum, but this procedure must be done in hospital after the woman has been assessed and ultrasound examination has excluded placenta praevia. If the haemorrhage is due to a benign local lesion it will be managed appropriately.

Fetal

A most unusual cause of antepartum haemorrhage in very late pregnancy is from fetal blood vessels. In rare cases the umbilical cord is inserted into the membranes in which the arteries and veins pass to reach the edge of the placenta. If by chance the placenta is also low lying the umbilical blood vessels pass over the internal os of the cervix (vasa praevia); when the membranes rupture the fetal vessels may tear and bleed. The blood is fetal and a small loss can lead to severe hypovolaemia of the fetus.

The presence of vasa praevia is difficult to diagnose but sometimes they can be suspected with colour Doppler ultrasonography. More usually the fetal heart rate may alter abruptly after membrane rupture accompanied by a very slight blood loss. Tests exist to differentiate fetal from maternal haemoglobin. The treatment must be a rapid caesarean section as the fetus cannot stand such blood loss for long.

Bleeding of unknown origin

The real cause of antepartum haemorrhage is unknown in a large number of women. They may have bled from separation of the lower part of a normally sited placental bed or the membranes may have sheared with tearing of very small blood vessels. Some placentas bleed early from their edge.

If the cause of antepartum haemorrhage is unknown the woman should not be dismissed lightly. The risk to her baby at subsequent labour is higher than background, although the risk to the mother does not seem to be great. It is good practice to keep such women in hospital, allowing them to return home if no further vaginal bleeding occurs after 10 days. This rule of thumb seems to cover most eventualities and so many women do not stay in hospital. Fetal growth should be monitored by ultrasonography. In labour, however, the fetus should be monitored for hypoxia: it is at higher risk than are babies whose mothers have not bled.

I thank Dr Rashmi Patel, St George's Hospital Medical School, for the ultrasound picture of placental abruption, and Mr Malcolm Pearce, St George's Hospital Medical School, for that of placenta praevia. The distribution of antepartum haemorrhage by type is reproduced by permission of Butterworth Heinemann from *British Births 1970* by R Chamberlain and G Chamberlain. The figure showing the cascade of events leading to disseminated intravascular coagulopathy is reproduced by permission of Churchill Livingstone from *Obstetrics* edited by A Turnbull and G Chamberlain.

Recommended reading
Barron SL. Antepartum haemorrhage. In: Turnbull A, Chamberlain G, eds. *Obstetrics*. London: Churchill Livingstone, 1989: 469-82.

SMALL FOR GESTATIONAL AGE

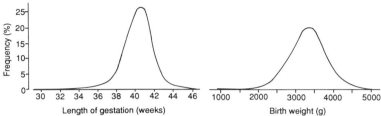

Distribution of length of gestation and birth weight (singletons, last menstrual period certain).

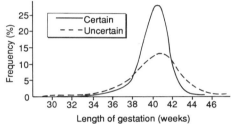

Distribution of length of gestation by knowledge of last menstrual period (singletons).

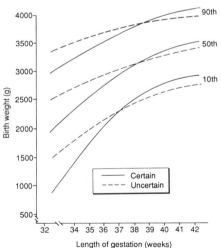

Centiles of birth weight by length of gestation and certainty of last menstrual period (singletons).

The problems of small babies and of preterm labour often go together and are the major causes of perinatal mortality and morbidity. Furthermore, they use up large amounts of facilities, manpower, and finance. Preterm labour is considered in the next chapter and the antenatal care of fetuses that are small for gestational age and of their mothers in this one.

The diagnosis of a small fetus is made more specific by examining the ratio of birth weight (or estimated birth weight) to gestational age. Both these measures have inherent problems.

Obstetricians estimate fetal weight either clinically or from measuring ultrasound determined diameters of the fetus in utero. Gestational age is derived from the mother's menstrual dates, which are usually confirmed by an ultrasound scan measuring the biparietal diameter performed before 20 weeks. In the National Birthday Trust's British Births Survey (1970) of 16 797 women only 13 634 (81·1%) were sure of their dates. The figure shows the distribution of length of gestation for women according to whether they were sure of their dates. The frequency of heavier babies was increased among those uncertain of the date of their last menstrual period. All women with unsure dates should have gestational age established by ultrasonography, as should those in whom there is a discrepancy between the dates derived from the last menstrual period and fetal size in early pregnancy. Obstetricians consider a baby to be small for gestational age when abdominal circumference readings fall below the second standard deviation of the mean; this is approximately the 2·3rd centile on serial ultrasonography.

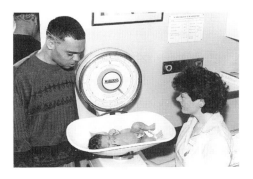

After birth paediatricians can weigh the baby and so have a more precise measure, although even this varies slightly with the conditions of weighing and when it is done. Gestational age is obtained from the obstetrician by one of the previously mentioned measures or from Dubowitz scoring. The data are plotted on a specific centile chart; various groups of paediatricians take small for gestational age as being below the 10th, the fifth, or the third centile. It is very important when examining data to know which of these measures was used. The 10th centile is rather crude and will include many babies whose growth has not actually been affected by placental bed disease.

Small for gestational age

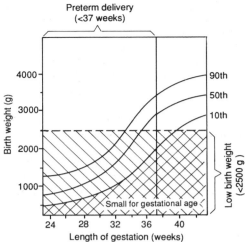

The relation between preterm and low birth weight babies. Babies who are small for gestational age fall under the 10th centile.

Causes

Much simpler was the old fashioned measure of prematurity taking a cut off point of a birth weight of less than 2500 g. Unfortunately, this includes small babies whose birth weight is appropriate for their gestational age and those who are small for their gestational age, two very different groups in clinical medicine. For example, babies born with a birth weight below 2500 g make up about 7% of the newborn population in the United Kingdom, about 3% in Sweden, and almost 11% in Hungary. Such mixed data would make a nonsense of studying the influences on fetal growth and so the definition of small for gestational age relating birth weight to length of intrauterine life stands for the moment.

In the United Kingdom most of the energy required by a pregnant woman can come from an ordinary diet, with little need for supplementation

---

Genetic abnormalities

Genetic abnormalities are an identifiable but not very common factor causing growth retardation. Trisomy 21 is the commonest example, though osteogenesis imperfecta, Potter's syndrome, and anencephaly may all be associated with intrauterine growth retardation. Other congenital malformations not yet proved to have a chromosome component are commonly found in fetuses that are small for gestational age; among them are gastrointestinal abnormalities such as atresia of the duodenum, gastroschisis, and omphalocele.

Maternal nutrition

In the United Kingdom the effect of maternal nutrition on low birth weight is probably small. Extremes of starvation associated with small babies are rare in Britain. During a pregnancy about 80 000 kilocalories (335 MJ) of extra energy is required, of which 36 000 kilocalories (150 MJ) is for maintenance metabolism.[1] Much of this can come from the everyday diet, and among well nourished women requirements change little for the first 10 weeks of pregnancy. Thence requirements gradually increase, but ordinary variations in food intake are unlikely to affect events. It is unwise to recommend that a mother eat for two in order to produce a larger baby as there are many covariables in nutrition other than what she eats and the most likely result is probably maternal obesity.

Intrauterine infection

Most intrauterine infections are viral or bacterial. Some 60% of babies with congenital rubella are born below the 10th centile of weight for gestation. Cytomegalovirus and toxoplasmosis (much less common in this country than in Europe) are associated with growth retardation in about 40% of affected infants. Malaria, ubiquitous in many tropical countries, causes a massive accumulation of monocytes in the intravillus space, which can lead to a fetus being small for gestational age. Syphilis, a rare disease in this country, used to be associated with babies being small for gestational age but the few babies now born with congenital syphilis do not exhibit this notably.

Drugs

Drugs may be a cause of babies being small for gestational age. The commonest cases in the United Kingdom are the results of burning tobacco, fumes being absorbed during cigarette smoking. The association between smoking and small for gestational age babies is well documented. The number of affected babies whose growth drops below the 10th centile increases during the last weeks of gestation.

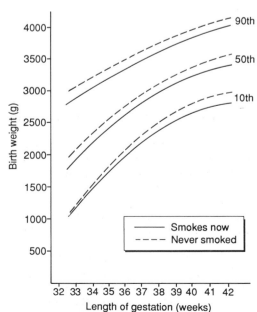

Centiles of birth weight by length of gestation and mother's smoking habit (singletons, last menstrual period certain).

The effect of alcohol is difficult to sort out. At the extreme end of the range, women drinking more than 45 units of alcohol a week, many babies are born with the fetal alcohol syndrome and a distinctly reduced birth weight. At lower intakes of alcohol covariables come into play; a deficient maternal diet and increased cigarette smoking are two well known ones.

In some studies multivariant analyses show that the main causal factor associated with low birth weight is not alcohol intake but cigarette smoking. The whole lifestyle is probably the important factor. Some doctors consider that smoking in pregnancy is the most important single cause of low birth weight, which is the greatest cause of death and illness in the first weeks of life.

The intake of narcotic drugs is commonly associated with low birth weight but, again, the total lifestyle of the woman may be the real factor. For this reason, perhaps, an increased incidence of small for gestational age babies persists with methadone users.

Therapeutic drugs such as carbamazepine and the valproates have been associated with an increased incidence of small for gestational age babies, as have the more powerful antiviral drugs such as azathioprine. Therapeutically powerful drugs are not given in pregnancy unless they are used to treat a serious maternal medical condition, which in itself may affect nutrition or metabolism of the mother and growth of the fetus.

Hypertension

One of the major current causes of babies being small for gestational age in the United Kingdom is hypertension in the mother, either pregnancy induced or pre-existing. After other features have been taken into account such types of hypertension are responsible for about a third of all cases of intrauterine growth retardation. The effects of hypertension are made worse when raised blood pressure is associated with proteinuria, implying a greater reduction of the maternal perfusion of the placental bed. The duration of the condition also has an effect—for example, 80% of mothers who have proteinuric pregnancy induced hypertension before the 34th week of pregnancy have infants with a birth weight below the 10th centile.

Other factors

The maternal body habitus is not a critical factor in babies being small for gestational age, but big women do produce larger children. The father's influence is less important, classically shown in the 1938 study of Walton and Hammond on Shire horses and Shetland ponies.[2]

The altitude at which a woman lives in pregnancy has an effect on fetal growth, particularly if she is not used to high altitudes.

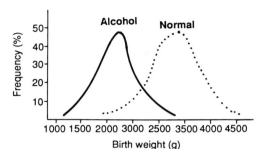

Distribution of birth weight in a normal population of women and in one consisting of women who drank more than 45 units of alcohol a week (heavy drinking).

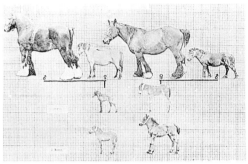

The effects of sire and mare on the size of offspring is shown in this 1938 experiment in which Shire horses and Shetland ponies were mated. The maternal influence predominates.

Diagnosis

- Symmetrical growth retardation occurs in low birthweight babies when the ratio of head to abdominal circumference is normal
- Asymmetrical growth retardation occurs in low birthweight babies when the ratio of head to abdominal circumference is increased

Extreme examples of fetuses that are severely small for gestational age can sometimes be diagnosed by palpation. This is most likely if the same observer sees the woman at each antenatal visit and uses the written records of previous visits longitudinally. In several control studies false positive rates as high as 50% and low predictive values have been found in the clinical estimation of intrauterine growth retardation.

Sometimes the lack of amniotic fluid is diagnosed more readily; oligohydramnios accompanies fetuses that are small for gestational age and therefore may lead observers to investigate more swiftly than when fetal size has been estimated clinically.

Most fetuses that are small for gestational age are diagnosed in this country by ultrasonography. When a good estimate of gestational age in early pregnancy has been obtained and fetal abnormalities have been excluded, ultrasound scans can give valid measures of fetal growth. Scans of the body area or circumference at the level of the umbilical vessels give a measure of liver growth. Another measure of somatic growth is femur length.

Small for gestational age

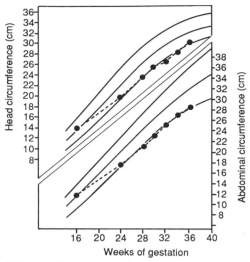

Ultrasound measures of the head and abdominal circumference. Although growth rates are diminished, they fall at the same rate—symmetrical growth retardation.

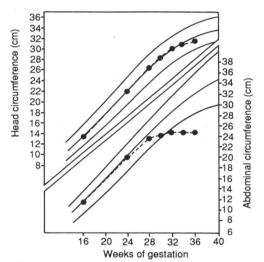

Ultrasound measures of head and abdominal circumference. Abdominal growth slows more than head growth—asymmetrical growth retardation.

Fetuses with small abdominal circumferences should have their head circumference measured and the ratio of head to abdominal circumference derived. A small for gestational age fetus with a normal ratio of head to abdominal circumference tends to be a perfect miniature (bonsai baby) and is often normal, representing the lower end of biological variation. Such fetuses, however, may also be associated with chromosomal anomalies, drugs, infection, and malnutrition.

Fetuses suffering from placental insufficiency tend to preserve growth of the head at the expense of the body because a protective mechanism shunts blood to the brain. Such babies suffer hypoxic and ischaemic brain damage in pregnancy before labour, but it may be only in labour that the fetal heart rate shows this.

Estimating fetal weight in utero uses one or more ultrasound measurements. All methods have a minimum error of 150 g/kg in relation to true fetal weight and are therefore better than clinical ways of predicting smaller babies.

Babies who are symmetrically small for gestational age (normal ratio of head to abdominal circumference) usually show normal growth subsequently and therefore only require serial ultrasound examination. Deciding which fetuses to examine karyometrically or for infection is difficult, but often an abnormal fetus will show minor structural markers such as cardiac defects, occipital fat pads, abnormal hand positions, or intracranial calcification. Asymmetrically small for gestational age fetuses used to be monitored by cardiotocography. Doppler studies of the uterine and umbilical circulation are rapidly replacing these (see chapter on checking for fetal wellbeing).

There is little help from assessing oestrogen concentrations in small for gestational age fetuses, although many obstetric departments have forgotten to stop using such tests. In an individual fetus longitudinal increases in plasma oestriol concentration are a reassuring sign, but the converse is not crisp enough to be a guide for action and positive predictive values are low (see chapter on checking for fetal wellbeing).

Small for gestational age fetuses may be screened by using early ultrasonography to confirm gestational age and later to confirm growth. Finer tuning is possible by Doppler measurement of the afferent blood supply to the placental bed, with later changes in blood velocity along the umbilical vessels giving a more precise warning of fetal state. In practice these are covered by an ultrasound reading of the biparietal diameter at 16-20 weeks to confirm gestation and a second scan of abdominal circumference at 32-36 weeks to check growth.

Mothers whose fetuses are at greater risk of intrauterine growth retardation often have several ultrasound readings performed in later pregnancy. Such women include those with a history of perinatal death and of intrauterine growth retardation as well as those in whom the fetus is exposed to some of the aetiological factors already considered and where oligohydramnios may give a clue.

Treatment

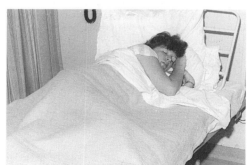

Woman lying in the left lateral position.

The ultimate treatment of a fetus with impaired growth associated with the placental bed is delivery. Diagnosis encapsulates the fact that a baby getting insufficient nutrition to grow at the expected rate will in labour be in greater danger of oxygen deprivation. Removal from the hostile environment would be the ultimate answer, but this might not be wise in early gestation (24-30 weeks); efforts are made to improve the blood supply to the placental bed.

Early work with abdominal decompression to improve uterine blood supply was unrewarding. Biopharmacological methods of increasing the diameter of the afferent vessels of the placental bed with β mimetics have been tried but have generally proved to be unsuccessful. The use of aspirin is currently under investigation in a multicentre trial (CLASP), and some general practitioners' patients may be a part of the study. Bed rest, particularly with the woman lying on her left side for some hours a day, should theoretically improve placental perfusion, but Doppler studies show little evidence for its effectiveness. Measures to restore the plasma volume and to give adequate hydration seem useful theoretically as they should decrease viscosity and lead to an improvement of intrauterine blood flow. Again, theory is not matched by practice.

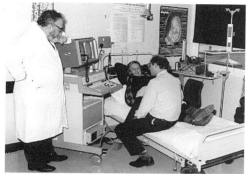

Corner of a fetal measurement laboratory.

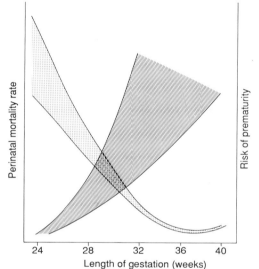

Perinatal mortality rate

Risk of prematurity

Length of gestation (weeks)

The relative risks to a fetus of staying in the uterus on the wrong side of a poor placental bed perfusion system ▨▨▨ compared with the risks of being delivered too soon ▨▨▨.

In fetuses that are symmetrically small for gestational age, correction and reversal of some of the causal factors might have helped, but it is too late to do this when the fetus is detectably small for gestational age. For example, curtailment of cigarette smoking should happen in early pregnancy. Such reduction in the first 16 weeks allows fetuses to follow a normal growth pattern rather than that of growth retarded babies of smoking mothers.

The mother of a fetus that is small for gestational age should attend a hospital with the capacity for more precise diagnosis and where special ultrasound and Doppler measurements are available. Many tertiary referral centres have a fetal measurement laboratory run on a day care basis. Women who live near large hospitals with such facilities can still be outpatients while having full surveillance. If they live away from the centre, however, they may have to be transferred and become inpatients; this is the keystone of the in utero transfer system widespread in the United Kingdom. Probably a third of the women admitted as in utero transfers have fetuses that are small for gestational age as their indication for admission.

The double ultrasonographic surveillance of fetal growth and placental bed blood flow allows a more precise assessment to be made of fetal progress. Prospective frequent and regular consultations with the neonatal paediatrician who will be involved is essential. The fetus must be delivered at the most appropriate time by the most appropriate method. The time depends on weighing up the risks of keeping the fetus inside the uterus— that is, those of diminished placental bed perfusion—against the risks of being outside—that is, the risks of immaturity and survival in a good intensive care neonatal unit. The critical gestational age for these decisions is being pushed back all the time; now the worrying time for most obstetricians and neonatal paediatricians is 24-28 weeks. Once a pregnancy passes 30 weeks the concern is much less, although the respiratory distress syndrome can still cause illness after delivery.

Conclusions

The diagnosis, causes, and management of small for gestational age fetuses are all still uncertain. The best management is prevention

It must be remembered that the definitions of small for gestational age are used imprecisely and much that was thought to be known about its causation depended on data that were not mutually comparable. Until Doppler measurement the measures of fetal wellbeing were also inexact; even Doppler ultrasonography is not the last word on the subject. The ultimate management depends on avoiding trouble. Maybe we are overprotective of fetuses that are small for gestational age, but it is the best that we can do in 1991.

The figures showing the distribution of birth weight, the distribution of the length of gestation, the centiles of birth weight by length of gestation and date of the last menstrual period, and the centiles of birth weight by length of gestation and maternal smoking habit are reproduced by permission of Butterworth Heinemann from *British Births 1970* by R Chamberlain and G Chamberlain; this is an account of the National Birthday Trust's 1970 study. I thank Mr Andrew Rolland of St George's Hospital Medical School for taking the photographs.

1 Hytten FE. Nutrition. In: Hytten FE, Chamberlain G, eds. *Clinical physiology in obstetrics.* 2nd ed. Oxford: Blackwell Scientific Publications, 1990:150-72.
2 Walton A, Hammond J. The maternal effects on growth in Shire horses and Shetland pony crosses. *Proc Roy Soc London [Biol]* 1938;**125**:311-35.

Recommended reading
Gluckman PD, Liggins GC. Regulation of fetal growth. In: Beard RW, Nathanielsz P, eds. *Fetal physiology and medicine.* New York: Marcel Dekker, 1984:511-58.

PRETERM LABOUR

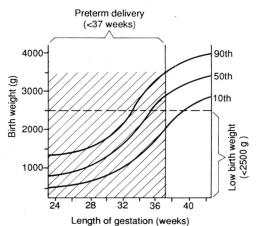

Relation between length of gestation and birth weight. Babies born in the crosshatched area are preterm irrespective of weight.

Preterm labour may result in the birth of an immature infant. Together with intrauterine growth retardation it is the main problem of obstetric care in the United Kingdom in the 1990s. The conventional definition of preterm labour includes women delivering before 37 completed weeks of gestation, but in practice in the United Kingdom problems arise mostly with births before 34 weeks. Babies more mature than this can be cared for successfully in many district general hospitals without intensive care facilities; most problems arise in babies weighing less than 1500 g (3·5 lb).

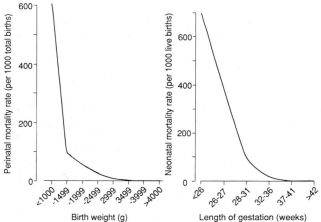

Birthweight specific perinatal mortality rates and gestation specific neonatal mortality rates for Scotland in 1988.

Perinatal mortality rates relate sharply to maturity and birth weight; similarly, neonatal mortality rates relate to gestational age at birth. Probably some 6% of babies in the United Kingdom are born before 37 weeks and 2% before the 32nd week of pregnancy.

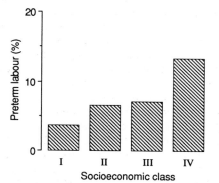

Relation between socioeconomic class and preterm labour among 12 000 pregnancies assessed prospectively.

Causes

Sociobiological background—The capacity for preterm labour is often predictable by a clustering of high risk factors. The mother's age, parity, and socioeconomic class bear strong associations with preterm labour. Socioeconomic class is an indicator of the woman's behaviour, nutrition, smoking, and previous medical and social existence. These may not be individual factors in their own right but are useful to identify women whose risk of preterm labour is increased.

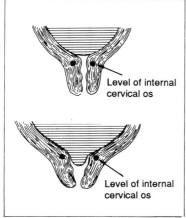

Cervical incompetence leads to a cone of unsupported membranes.

Reproductive history—A multiparous woman's obstetric history may give prognostic clues; the chances of a preterm delivery are tripled after one previous preterm birth and increased sixfold after two. These are two simple sets of risks; other outcomes bring in differential variables. Past studies have been diminished by not including the woman's total obstetric history, which needs careful consideration in the case of each woman.

Medical history—Recurrent lower urinary tract infections are not usually associated with recurrent preterm labour, although pyelonephritis may be. The renal tract should be investigated between pregnancies and reinfection prevented by prophylactic antibiotics in future pregnancies.

Effectiveness of cervical cerclage in reducing preterm delivery and rates of stillbirth, miscarriage, and neonatal death[1]

	No in group		Odds ratio and 95% confidence interval						
	Experimental	Control	0·01	0·1	0·5	1	2	10	100
Delivered:									
Before 33 weeks	59/454	82/451			●—				
Before 37 weeks	124/454	146/451			●—				
Stillbirth, miscarriage, or									
neonatal death	37/454	54/451			●				

Data analysed to 1988.

Uterine structural abnormalities can be a recurrent factor, the best documented being cervical incompetence. This follows damage or overstretch of the cervical internal os—an illformed muscular sphincter—and is a mechanical diagnosis first observed by obstetricians in the 1940s and made familiar by the work of Shirodkar and McDonald in the 1950s. The truer picture of the place of cervical incompetence and its management in preterm labour had to await a randomised controlled trial in the late 1980s run jointly by the Medical Research Council and the Royal College of Obstetricians and Gynaecologists; the results put into proportion the importance of cervical incompetence as an individual factor in preterm delivery.[1]

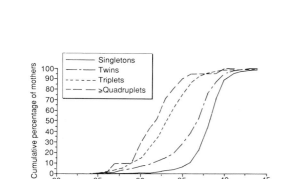

Cumulative gestational age at delivery for multiple pregnancies. By 37 weeks delivery has occurred in 97% of quadruplet, 96% of triplet, 55% of twin, and 25% of singleton pregnancies.

Complications of pregnancy—A twin pregnancy is a marker for preterm labour. The mean gestation of twins is 37 weeks and therefore many will be born before this time.

Several National Birthday Trust studies have shown the association of preterm labour with antepartum haemorrhage, irrespective of the cause of the bleeding.

An obvious but unusual factor associated with preterm labour is abdominal surgical intervention when appendicitis or a complication of an ovarian cyst may require surgical treatment. The woman may go into labour soon after the operation, but with modern anaesthesia most do not. Hard physical work in pregnancy is associated with preterm labour, particularly if it is repetitive and boring or in an unpleasant, noisy environment. This factor is discussed in the chapter on work in pregnancy.

Abnormalities of the fetus are often associated with preterm labour and there may also be polyhydramnios, which in itself can lead to premature membrane rupture and preterm labour.

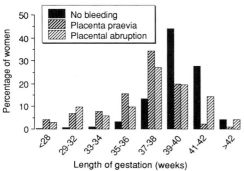

Time of delivery among women who had no vaginal bleeding in pregnancy compared with that among those with placenta praevia or placental abruption (n=17 005).[2]

Infection and premature membrane rupture—Infection of the lower uterus and the membranes is an important feature that is poorly investigated epidemiologically. The presence of micro-organisms in the membranes is associated with an increased production of prostaglandins, one of the main factors associated with the onset of labour. Proteases, coagulases, and elastases are also produced by invading micro-organisms, whose endotoxins may stimulate labour directly as well as through prostaglandin metabolism. Low grade chorioamnionitis (infection of the membranes) is much commoner after premature rupture of the membranes, when an ascending infection from the vagina may produce such biochemical changes. One of the commonest organisms is the β haemolytic streptococcus, which is found as a commensal in the vagina in about 5% of women but may be a cause of preterm labour in up to 20%. Premature membrane rupture itself is a commonly quoted cause of preterm labour; this may be due to the infection that weakened the forewaters or to the removal of the forewaters' mechanical support from the cervix.

Preterm labour

Induction—Preterm labour is also caused iatrogenically: labour is induced in about 15% of women in this country, though in some units the rate rises to 40%. Many of the inductions will obviously be in women after 37 weeks' gestation but some will be performed before this. The problem of rhesus incompatibility, previously a major indication, is reduced; in its place is pregnancy induced proteinuric hypertension and intrauterine growth retardation. Women with either of these problems should be delivered at hospitals that can cope with the neonatal sequelae of such inductions, which produce a large proportion of babies who are born well before the 37th week of pregnancy.

Prevention

The recognition of some of the triggers of preterm labour has led a few obstetricians to take action to prevent labour. There is little objective evidence that bed rest and the use of prophylactic tocolytic agents are helpful, although a doctor might use either of these managements to satisfy a mother who has previously undergone preterm labour and has faith in them. Repeated, carefully taken, high vaginal swabs to give the pattern of micro-organisms in the upper vagina may be useful. Should the organisms found be relevant—for example, β haemolytic streptococcus or listeria—active antibiotic treatment may eradicate colonisation and thus reduce the risks of preterm labour. This approach is under evaluation.

Several centres have used programmes during early and mid-pregnancy to educate women with a history of preterm delivery to try to prevent a recurrence of the problem. There is no easy method of doing this in a group; the success of such programmes depends on the individual woman and her individual attendants. All the factors discussed so far must be considered, and the woman should obviously try to avoid those which seem to be the more relevant in her case. Even with the most intensive antenatal education programmes, preterm deliveries are not cut to less than about 3·5%, a background rate in many populations. Success in this subject may come eventually after a conscious effort to modify the lifestyle, socioeconomic conditions, and medical problems of each individual patient.

Diagnosis—As with labour at term, diagnosing the onset of preterm labour is much easier retrospectively than at the time. You can look back and say a labour probably started at a certain time, but to do so prospectively is much harder. The general practitioner is left with the difficult task of deciding whether any group of uterine contractions will progress to cervical dilatation or whether they are just stronger Braxton Hicks contractions. The diagnosis may be assisted by external tocographic measurement of uterine contractions with a semiquantitative external monitor. Any woman thought to be in preterm labour should go to the local maternity unit as soon as possible for further assessment. There tocography may help, and assessment of the cervix may be valuable. About half of the women who present with regular, painful contractions will not progress to labour.

If preterm labour seems inevitable, treatment may be given to postpone it. Otherwise, the woman may be kept in for 24 hours to see if labour follows; if not, she can be discharged home to the care of her general practitioner. It is easy to be wise after the event, but only by sending every woman about whom there is reasonable doubt to the maternity unit will clinicians not miss the occasional woman who goes into very early preterm labour.

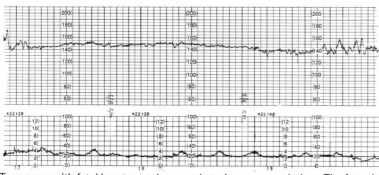

Tocogram with fetal heart rate above and uterine pressure below. The fetus is asleep for much of this trace, although regular small contractions of the uterus are seen.

Before 32 weeks' gestation short term inhibition of labour allows:
- Transfer to the delivery unit best equipped for special neonatal care
- Steroids to be given to help mature the fetal respiratory system

Inhibition of established preterm labour

If a woman is in real preterm labour a decision has to be made whether labour should be stopped. It is probably wise not to do so if the mother's blood pressure is greatly raised, there is proved infection in the endocervical or decidual regions, or the fetus has a lethal abnormality. Some obstetricians would consider further that it was unwise to inhibit labour in the presence of long term rupture of the membranes, severe intrauterine growth retardation, or an antepartum haemorrhage. Each of these cases must be decided on their own merits.

Other than these exceptions, in most cases before 28 weeks it is worth trying to stop preterm labour to buy intrauterine time for the fetus. In the short term this can allow emergency treatment such as steroids to help maturation of the fetal respiratory system or allow transfer of the woman to a centre with better neonatal care facilities for a very small baby after delivery. These decisions must be made in consultation with the paediatricians as the practical management of any baby resulting from a preterm labour will depend on their skills and facilities. In a large well equipped obstetric-paediatric unit the borderline comes at about 28 weeks, provided that all other features of the pregnancy are normal.

If it is considered necessary to stop preterm labour a range of agents exist. Alcohol and the progestogens are obsolete. Prostaglandin synthesis inhibitors (such as indomethacin) are effective but may have side effects in mother and fetus. Calcium antagonists are currently undergoing trial. The main agents in current use are β agonists, of which the commonest two in the United Kingdom are ritodrine and salbutamol. These drugs work equally well on the myometrial cells and may postpone labour for a time. There is little evidence from meta-analyses of many studies that they reduce either perinatal mortality rates or postponement of labour over a long period.[3] Their use will depend on the ripeness of the cervix—the less ripe the more likely that action will be effective. They are best used before 32 weeks of pregnancy and probably work better in the absence of infection. Though little evidence shows that prophylactic oral β mimetic agents prevent preterm labour, oral maintenance after intravenous inhibition has some effect.

Ritodrine and salbutamol have side effects, the most noticeable being tachycardia felt as palpitations in the neck; they may also be associated with mild sweating and headache. Rare cases of pulmonary oedema have been reported, and it is essential to watch the woman's fluid intake if the tocolytic agent is being given intravenously. Some have reported fetal macrosomia after long term use of β agonists, but this is unusual. They are better not used or used only with extreme caution in women with cardiac disease, hyperthyroidism, or diabetes.

Effectiveness of β mimetic tocolytics used in preterm labour in reducing perinatal death. The numbers are the proportions of perinatal deaths[3]

Study	No in group Experimental	Control	Odds ratio and 95% confidence interval
Christensen et al (1980)	1/14	0/16	
Spellacy et al (1979)	1/15	4/15	
Barden (unpublished)	1/12	0/13	
Hobel (unpublished)	2/17	0/16	
Cotton et al (1984)	1/19	4/19	
Howard et al (1982)	1/16	1/21	
Ingemarsson (1976)	0/15	0/15	
Larsen et al (1986)	1/49	2/50	
Calder and Patel (1985)	0/37	1/39	
Scommegna (unpublished)	0/16	1/17	
Mariona (unpublished)	1/4	1/5	
Wesselius-De Casparis et al (1971)	2/33	1/30	
Leveno et al (1986)	2/56	3/55	
Larsen et al (1980)	11/131	2/45	
Adam (1966)	9/28	7/24	
Typical odds ratio and 95% confidence interval			

Effectiveness of β mimetic tocolytics used in preterm labour in reducing preterm delivery. The numbers are the proportions of women delivering before 37 weeks[3]

Study	No in group Experimental	Control	Odds ratio and 95% confidence interval
Christensen et al (1980)	14/14	16/16	
Spellacy et al (1979)	12/14	13/15	
Barden (unpublished)	6/12	13/13	
Hobel (unpublished)	10/16	8/15	
Cotton et al (1984)	15/19	16/19	
Howard et al (1982)	9/15	5/18	
Ingemarsson (1976)	3/15	12/15	
Larsen et al (1986)	14/49	23/50	
Calder and Patel (1985)	23/37	19/39	
Scommegna (unpublished)	10/15	10/16	
Mariona (unpublished)	3/4	3/5	
Wesselius-De Casparis et al (1971)	13/33	21/30	
Leveno et al (1986)	40/54	42/52	
Larsen et al (1980)	65/131	21/45	
Sivasamboo (1972)	14/33	20/32	
Typical odds ratio and 95% confidence interval			

Note the small numbers and wide confidence intervals in some of the studies in these two meta-analyses

Once treatment with β agonists has been started, the next decision is where the woman is to deliver if labour proceeds. If the unit cannot cope with very small babies, in utero transfer must be considered. The woman should be sent to a tertiary referral centre in the region that can manage babies of this degree of immaturity. The alternative philosophy is to allow the baby to be delivered in the peripheral centre and, if necessary, transfer the child to the tertiary referral unit by ex utero transfer. There is much debate in the United Kingdom currently about which of these is more effective. In utero transfer may not be necessary every time; it is used as a precaution but it allows the woman to be in the tertiary referral centre that is able to provide more sophisticated obstetric as well as neonatal care—for example, Doppler flow studies. Ex utero transfer allows the woman to stay closer to her home at the local hospital she has chosen. However, specialist antenatal tests may not be available, obstetricians may not be as experienced in the delivery of very small babies, and expert paediatricians may not be available at the time of delivery because of the many other calls on obstetricians' and paediatricians' time. In addition, with road traffic conditions in the United Kingdom there is no guarantee that help can get to even the nearest district hospital quickly. At present the philosophy is in favour of in utero transfer, but it may not stay so for long in the reorganised NHS.

Expert care for babies expected to be very small
- In utero transfer to obstetric/neonatal referral centre
- Delivery in district general hospital and ex utero transfer to specialist centre

---

Conclusions

Preterm labour and small for gestational age fetuses constitute the most serious current problems in obstetrics

---

This chapter and the previous one are concerned with the most serious problems of current obstetrics. Getting the best results for very small babies is the most hopeful line of advance for the 1990s. It needs coordination from family doctors, obstetricians, midwives, and neonatal paediatricians with individual treatments tailored to individual mothers.

The data for perinatal and neonatal mortality rates for Scotland are taken from the Scottish stillbirths and neonatal deaths report of 1989 produced by the Information Office of the Scottish Health Service. The figure showing the cumulative distribution of singleton and multiple births is reproduced by permission of the Office of Population Censuses and Surveys from *Three, Four and More*, published by HMSO.

1 MRC/RCOG Working Party on Cervical Cerclage. Interim report of the Medical Research Council/Royal College of Obstetricians and Gynaecologists multicentre randomised trial of cervical cerclage. *Br J Obstet Gynaecol* 1988;**95**:437-45.
2 Chamberlain G, Phillip E, Howlett B, Masters K. In: Chamberlain R, Chamberlain G, eds. *British births 1970*. London: Heinemann, 1976.
3 Chambers I, Enkin M, Keirse MJNC, eds. *Effective care in pregnancy and childbirth*. Vol 2. *Childbirth*. Oxford: Oxford University Press, 1989: 705, 707.

Recommended reading
Yu VYH, Wood EC, eds. *Prematurity*. London: Churchill Livingstone, 1987.

MULTIPLE PREGNANCY

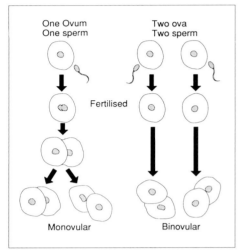

Monovular and binovular twins.

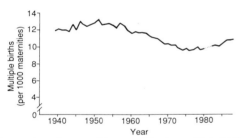

Proportion of maternities resulting in multiple births (England and Wales, 1939-89).

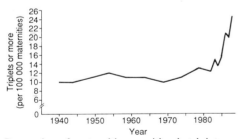

Proportion of maternities resulting in triplet or higher order birth (England and Wales, 1939-89).

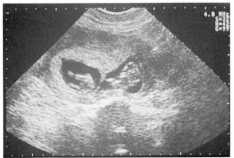

In early pregnancy twin sacs and embryos can be shown by ultrasonography.

Multiple pregnancy is a mixed blessing. On the one hand is the instant family, on the other are the increased perinatal mortality and morbidity as well as a much greater load for the mother after delivery.

Types

Multiple pregnancy follows either the division of an oocyte fertilised by one sperm into two separate bodies (identical or monozygotic twins) or the fertilisation of more than one egg by separate sperm (non-identical or dizygotic twins). In higher multiple pregnancies than twins a combination of these two mechanisms happens.

In uniovular twins division into two separate bodies was thought to occur only at a very early stage but it can in fact take place up to several days after fertilisation.

Prevalence

The prevalence of twin births in the United Kingdom is one in 105 deliveries, of triplets one in 10 000, and of quadruplets about one in every half a million deliveries. There is a natural variation between races; Japanese women have one of the lowest rate of twins and those from some African countries have a much higher rate, up to one in 30 deliveries. Multiple pregnancies also increase with maternal age. These biological variations are due to an increase in the dizygotic twinning rates, based on the capacity of the woman to produce more than one oocyte at the time of ovulation.

The prevalence of multiple pregnancy has been increasing in the United Kingdom in the past decade. For higher multiples than twins the rate doubled from 12 per 100 000 to 29 per 100 000 between 1980 and 1989. Though a part of this is due to the increasing number of mothers over 35, the iatrogenic effect of ovarian stimulation and in vitro fertilisation programmes are also important. Concern about this has led bodies such as the Interim Licensing Authority (which became the Human Fertilisation and Embryology Authority) to make recommendations about the maximum number of oocytes or embryos transferred at assisted fertilisation.

Diagnosis

Twin pregnancies used to be diagnosed clinically when the woman reported her symptoms of pregnancy were worse than usual and the uterus was found to be bigger than would be expected from gestational dates (after about 24 weeks); sometimes twins were diagnosed for the first time in labour. Often the fetal parts are hard to determine but palpation of more than two poles is suggestive of twins. Now in the United Kingdom most women have an ultrasound scan at 16 to 20 weeks and so multiple pregnancies are usually diagnosed much sooner. In the Scottish twin survey 70% of multiple pregnancies were diagnosed by ultrasonography before 20 weeks and 95% were diagnosed in the antenatal period. When a twin pregnancy is diagnosed by ultrasonography the increased incidence of congenital abnormalities should be remembered and a thorough ultrasound examination of each fetus performed between 20 and 24 weeks.

Problems

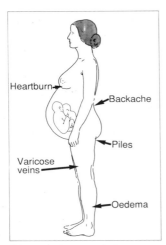

Changes that may follow an overdisteded uterus.

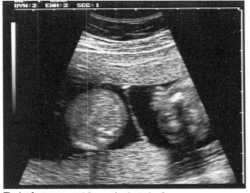

Twin fetuses at 16 weeks just before amniocentesis. Twin sacs are easily seen.

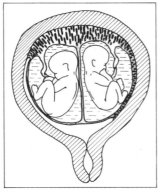

The greater area of placental implantation on the left of the uterus means that it may encroach on the lower segment.

The increased uterine size leads to greater pressure on venous return. The frequency of the group of conditions that male obstetricians call minor problems (for example, varicose veins in the leg) is increased. Furthermore, the woman may have more symptoms of nausea in early pregnancy associated with the higher human chorionic gonadotrophin concentrations.

Congenital abnormalities

Many congenital abnormalities are more frequent in twin births. Neural tube defects, heart abnormalities, and the incidences of Turner's and Klinefelter's syndromes are all increased. About twice as many live births from multiple pregnancies have a major congenital abnormality compared with singleton pregnancies.

Some of these abnormalities may be detected by ultrasonography, others require amniocentesis. In multiple pregnancy this test is associated with a 3% rate of miscarriage compared with about 0·5% in singleton pregnancies. Care must be taken to identify the fluid from each sac as the abnormality may be in one fetus only. Should severe abnormality be found in one fetus of a multiple pregnancy with two sacs the obstetrician may consider that the normal fetus is at increased risk and recommend selective fetocide. This can be by cardiac puncture, injection of air into the umbilical vein, or intravenous injection of potassium chloride. Such management should be at a regional centre well used not just to performing these procedures but to the very important counselling that goes on before and after such an event. The risk of preterm labour in the unaffected pregnancy is increased.

Pregnancy induced hypertension

The incidence of pregnancy induced hypertension is greatly increased in multiple pregnancies and eclampsia is also commoner. Increased antenatal vigilance is needed and some obstetricians advocate prophylactic bed rest. Antihypertensive treatment should be used as in any other pregnancy complicated by proteinuric hypertension (see chapter on raised blood pressure in pregnancy), and the ultimate treatment of delivery may be required earlier than for singletons, a more difficult decision as preterm twins fare less well than do preterm singletons. A caesarean section is more frequently needed.

Anaemia

Commonly anaemia is reported as being more frequent in multiple than in singleton pregnancies. Some of this is due to the greater expansion in blood volume in women with twins whereby the plasma increases more than the red cell bulk, so lowering the haemoglobin concentration. If the mean corpuscular haemoglobin concentration is used as a measure of anaemia, anaemia is not more frequent in multiple pregnancies than in singletons provided that adequate nutrition and iron intake are maintained. Greater demands of the growing fetuses for folate have led to some reports of megaloblastic anaemia so folate supplements are commonly given.

Antepartum haemorrhage

Antepartum haemorrhage would be thought to be commoner in multiple pregnancy because of the greater surface area of the placental bed. The Aberdeen twin data set showed rates of antepartum haemorrhage in twin pregnancies to be 6% compared with 4·7% in singleton pregnancies ($p = <0·05$). Much of this difference, however, was made up of antepartum haemorrhage from unknown origin; only a few were caused by placental abruption or placenta praevia.

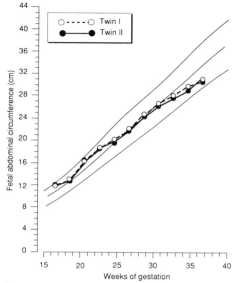

Growth of non-identical twins through pregnancy set against the mean (2SD) singleton growth curve.

Intrauterine growth retardation

The growth of each fetus in multiple pregnancies mirrors that of the singleton until about 24 weeks of gestation; thence growth rates for most twins are still as for singletons but occasionally one or both may show a decrease. This is difficult to detect on clinical examination for polyhydramnios may cause imprecision in estimation of fetal size. Repeated symphysiofundal height measurements can give a clue, particularly when both babies have retarded growth. Repeated ultrasound estimations of fetal size are the most useful way to check growth by plotting measurements of individual fetuses longitudinally through pregnancy. These data are not very different from the standard head or abdomen growth curves from singleton pregnancies until the last weeks. The estimation of fetal weight by various formulas based on the diameters of the fetus are not as useful in twin pregnancies as in the singleton as the fetus is often more flexed and its head more frequently dolichocephalic, resulting in an unrepresentative biparietal measurement. Discordance between the growth of a pair of fetuses should warn the obstetrician of the possibility of twin to twin transfusion. This is more common in monochorionic twins.

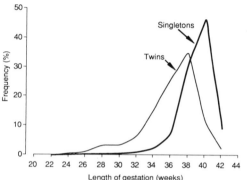

Percentage frequency distribution of length of gestation for singleton and twin pregnancies.

Preterm labour

The median gestation for human singleton pregnancy is just over 40 weeks whereas that for twins is 37 weeks and that for triplets about 33 weeks. The commonest single cause of perinatal mortality in multiple pregnancies is low birth weight. Though intrauterine growth retardation might also be present, birth weight is low mostly because of a preterm delivery. A measure of this problem is seen in the 30% of all liveborn triplets and 60% of liveborn quadruplets who have to stay in a neonatal intensive care unit for more than a month after delivery. The incidence of preterm labour (before 37 weeks) in twin pregnancies ranges from 20% to 50% compared with from 5% to 10% in singleton pregnancies.

An important part of antental care for multiple pregnancy is trying to detect those women who are likely to go into early preterm labour and prevent this if possible; if not, ensure that they are delivered in the correct surroundings to look after immature babies. Some obstetricians find the examination of the cervix routinely from 28 weeks gives a clue to its increasing ripeness (length, firmness, and dilatation). This seems to be of more use in primiparous than multiparous women. Others assess the cervix with ultrasonography, endeavouring to predict early labour.

An essential element lies in informing the mother; antenatal education of women with twins must devote a large proportion of time to the signs of early preterm labour.

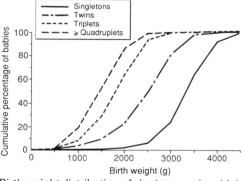

Birth weight distribution of singleton and multiple births.

The greater stretch of the myometrium imposed by multiple pregnancy increases the risk of preterm labour and several measures have been tried in the antenatal period to prevent this. Sympathomimetic drugs such as ritodrine have been given prophylactically, but most controlled trials have shown no benefit of this in twin pregnancy. Cervical cerclage inserted when a twin pregnancy is diagnosed does not seem to confer any increased benefits. Some consider that coitus may tip the balance in a woman who is on the edge of going into preterm labour, because of both the mechanical stimulation and the release into the vagina of prostaglandin rich fluid. The avoidance of coitus by women with twin pregnancies, however, does not seem to be associated with any significant prolongation of gestation.

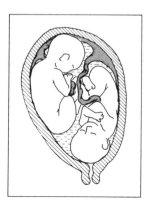

The extra stretch that twins place on the myometrium usually ensures that labour starts well before term.

Management

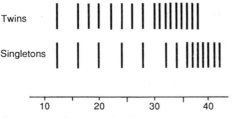

Twins

Singletons

10   20   30   40

Frequency of antenatal visits.

Antenatal care of a woman with a multiple pregnancy needs more vigilance than that of a woman with a singleton pregnancy. The woman with a multiple pregnancy will need more social support and advice for she is embarking on an extra load before, during, and after delivery. Her socioeconomic state and its implications should be explored. She needs to be seen more often and will require more investigations. Care can still be shared with the general practitioner in early pregnancy but after about 24 weeks many obstetricians would prefer the care to be where tests can take place—the hospital antenatal clinic.

Prenatal diagnosis in multiple pregnancy needs careful counselling. All twins should have a detailed ultrasound scan for anomalies at 18-20 weeks and preferably a detailed fetal cardiac scan at 22-24 weeks. At least monthly ultrasound scans should be performed to monitor fetal growth.

Blood pressure and urinary protein concentration are checked at each clinic, as is the symphysiofundal height. Palpation is performed by an experienced doctor or midwife, and from 30 weeks in many centres the cervix is checked regularly.

Management of twin pregnancy

- Antenatal care at hospital clinic after 24 weeks
- Detailed ultrasound scan for abnormalities at 18-20 weeks
- Fetal cardiac scan at 21-24 weeks
- Monthly ultrasound scans to monitor fetal growth
- ? Cervix checked regularly after 30 weeks
- More frequent antenatal visits
- Instruction of mother on symptoms of preterm labour
- Possible admission to hospital for rest

Because of the increased risk of pregnancy induced hypertension, women carrying twins were traditionally admitted to hospital from 32 weeks to ensure bed rest. The other justification for this was postponed preterm labour and so prolonged pregnancy. It is now realised that antenatal time in bed in hospital is not always the best rest: home is more relaxing. Furthermore, it would be more logical to bring the woman into hospital from 24 to 30 weeks, rather than at a later stage of pregnancy. Neither of the desirable aims has been fulfilled in randomised controlled trials of hospital admission after 32 weeks. Though reports from previous decades seemed to show a benefit in one or other of these aims (preventing raised blood pressure or postponing early labour), truly randomised studies in the 1980s have been unable to show benefit. When the disadvantages of separating the woman from her household, as well as the cost to society, are considered, the disadvantages of a routine policy of hospital admission outweigh the advantages. A woman should be advised, however, to come into hospital at a much lower critical level if, in her individual case, specific symptoms arise. These might include the development of hypertension or the threat of early preterm labour. The woman should be made well aware of the warning signs of preterm labour (see previous chapter) and be encouraged to act on a low level of suspicion.

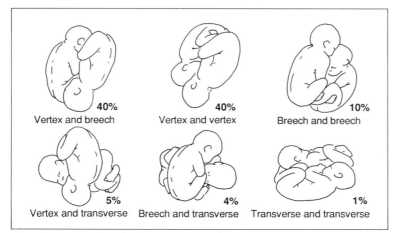

40%
Vertex and breech

40%
Vertex and vertex

10%
Breech and breech

5%
Vertex and transverse

4%
Breech and transverse

1%
Transverse and transverse

Lie and presentation of twins at the start of labour.

The exact lie and presentation of each twin is often difficult to determine in the last weeks of pregnancy. In many ways detail is not vital but the general practitioner should ensure that the leading twin is longitudinal. Nearly always the head or a breech is the lower presenting part. In cases of doubt a vaginal examination will usually give a clearer idea for if a presenting part is in or above the pelvis it can be identified more easily by the vaginal finger than through the abdominal wall. Ultrasonography or radiography may be needed for confirmation of the fetal lies and presentations.

Outcome

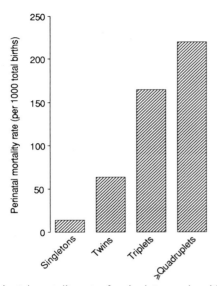

Perinatal mortality rates for singleton and multiple pregnancies (England and Wales, 1975-86 but excluding 1981).

Multiple pregnancies have increased risks for both mother and fetuses. Perinatal mortality rates are about four times higher among twins than singletons, being higher still among monozygotic twins. Rates are even greater in triplets and quadruplets. About three quarters of the increased mortality is caused by immaturity following preterm delivery, by intrauterine growth retardation, or by some combination of the two. The perinatal mortality rate for the second twin at vaginal deliveries is much higher than that of the first, depending on the skills of the doctor in charge of the delivery. The perinatal mortality rates associated with antepartum haemorrhage, premature rupture of the membranes, and proteinuric hypertension are increased.

Though some of the increased perinatal mortality rate in twins can be reduced by careful delivery, a large component can be helped by good antenatal care. This includes diagnosing the multiple pregnancy early, carefully managing the woman throughout pregnancy, and either postponing early preterm labour or ensuring that it takes place in an appropriate unit with a good neonatal unit.

The figures showing the proportions of maternities resulting in multiple births are reproduced by permission of the Office of Population Censuses and Surveys from *Three, Four and More*, published by HMSO, and based on data from OPCS Birth Statistics (series FM1) and the figure showing the frequency of birth weights of babies from singleton and multiple births is also reproduced with permission from *Three, Four and More*.

Recommended reading
MacGillivray I, Campbell D, Thompson B. *Twins and twinning*. Chichester: Wiley, 1988.
Botting B, MacFarlane A, Price F. *Three, four, and more — a study of triplets and higher order births*. London: HMSO, 1990.

VITAL STATISTICS OF BIRTH

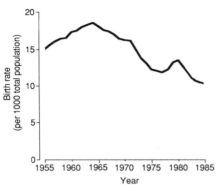

Birth rates in England and Wales, 1955-84.

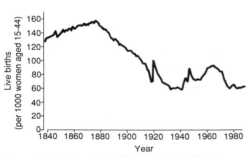

General fertility rates in England and Wales, 1840-1988.

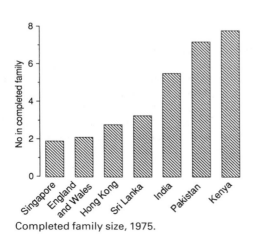

Completed family size, 1975.

Doctors are mostly literate but are commonly innumerate. We are largely ignorant and frightened of the safe and helpful use of figures because we have never been taught to understand them properly. In consequence we often try to dismiss them, believing that they are used during medical debate in a biased fashion to support the arguments of the proponents but are put to one side as non-relevant or non-significant by the opponents. This is a head in the sand attitude as statistics are extremely helpful in providing evidence of changes. Obstetricians are in fact well used to monitoring their activities statistically, having collected and published data long before the current fashion for audit started.

To be useful medical statistics must be
- Collected properly from a prescribed population
- Analysed in a valid fashion so as not to produce bias
- Presented promptly in a digestible, unbiased form.

In the United Kingdom these three criteria have been met by the national statutory handling of data on births, perinatal deaths, and maternal deaths. District registrars refer data centrally to the registrars general of the four kingdoms; checking, analysis, and comment on final data come from the Office of Population Censuses and Surveys in London and from equivalent departments in Wales, Scotland, and Northern Ireland. The Scottish system currently gives the most speedy and best produced information.

Birth rates

The number of babies born is counted by two processes, birth registration and birth notification. These are two statutory obligations—registration on parents, notification on professional staff.

Birth rates are often expressed as a ratio of the number of births to the number of people in the existing population, usually gathered from the decennial census.

$$\text{Birth rate} = \frac{\text{No of births} \times 1000}{\text{No of people in the population}}$$

The birth rate in the United Kingdom in 1988 was 7·3 per 1000.

The denominator in the birth rate formula includes, however, men, who never give birth, and women under 15 and over 44, who are mostly outside the reproductive age group. Hence the denominator does not relate to the numerator very well; an alternative measure is more commonly used in the Western world.

$$\text{General fertility rate} = \frac{\text{No of babies born} \times 1000}{\text{No of women in the population aged 15-44}}$$

The general fertility rate in the United Kingdom in 1985-7 was 62 per 1000. International comparisons are harder because only countries with good census systems can break down population data to determine the number of women aged 15-44.

For the less numerically minded, completed family size is a user friendly statistic: we can all imagine the size of a family. Unfortunately, these data depend on uncertain estimates and are usually produced some years after the women concerned have passed their reproductive years and completed their family. Obviously, to increase any population the number in a family needs to be more than two. In much of western Europe it is 1·7 to 2·2, whereas in Kenya it is 7·8, showing a rapidly increasing population.

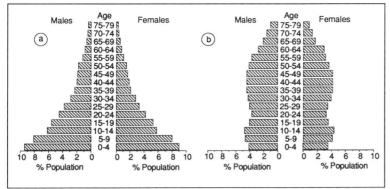

The shifts in population over the years can be shown by demograms that group the population in five or 10 year age bands. Thus the effects of past events can be seen; some idea of the future makeup of a population can also be predicted and future needs in society such as schools, colleges, and the numbers of people in any age group who are available for jobs can be forecast.

Demogram of (a) a rapidly developing country and (b) a developed country.

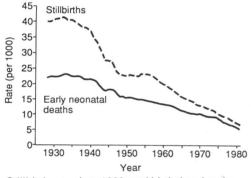

Stillbirth rates (per 1000 total births) and early neonatal death rates (per 1000 live births) in England and Wales, 1930-80. From 1935 the stillbirth rate has fallen more than that of neonatal deaths. From 1975 they have been parallel because of the decline in neonatal deaths.

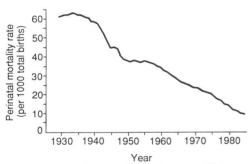

Perinatal mortality rates in England and Wales, 1930-85.

Perinatal mortality

Deaths of babies around the time of birth are assessed by three sets of statistics.

(1) Stillbirths or late intrauterine deaths occur when a child is delivered after the 28th completed week of pregnancy but shows no signs of life at birth:

$$\text{Stillbirth rate} = \frac{\text{No of babies born dead after 28 weeks} \times 1000}{\text{Total births (live and stillborn)}}$$

(2) Neonatal death is recorded when babies who are born alive (regardless of gestation) die in the first 28 days of life; early neonatal deaths refer to babies who die in the first seven days after birth. All babies who die in the first year of life are recorded as infant deaths but those who die after the first four weeks are defined as postneonatal deaths.

$$\text{Neonatal death rate} = \frac{\text{No of babies dying between 1-28 days} \times 1000}{\text{No of live births}}$$

(3) In the past 50 years perinatal mortality rates have been used to group together all babies whose deaths may have some relation to obstetric events; thus all stillbirths and neonatal deaths in the first week after birth are considered.

$$\text{Perinatal mortality rate} = \frac{\text{Stillbirths + neonatal deaths in the first 7 days} \times 1000}{\text{Total births (live and stillborn)}}$$

The perinatal mortality rate in England and Wales in 1990 was 8·3 per 1000 total births.

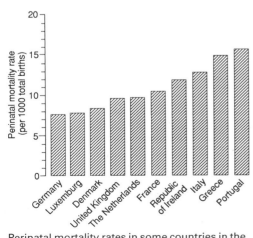

Perinatal mortality rates in some countries in the European Community.

There is some degree of dissatisfaction with the use of perinatal mortality rates as an index of obstetric performance. Many babies born before 28 weeks of gestation now survive in neonatal units. Others with congenital lethal malformations may be kept alive in such units until the second or third week and so are not included in the perinatal mortality rate. We may return to looking at stillbirth rates (possibly changing definitions of viability to 24 weeks' gestation in England, Wales, and Scotland) and neonatal death rates as separate statistics.

Vital statistics of birth

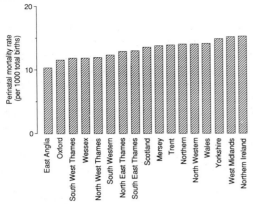

Perinatal mortality rates in the English regional health authorities and in Wales, Scotland, and Northern Ireland, 1976-87.

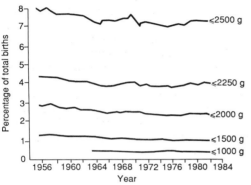

The proportions of babies in different birthweight bands has altered little in the past 30 years.

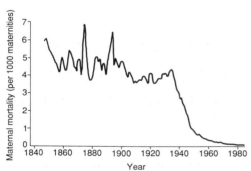

Maternal mortality in England and Wales, 1845-1984.

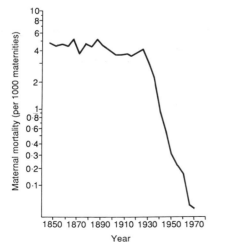

Maternal mortality in England and Wales, 1850-1970, plotted on a semi-log scale to show the continued decline in the past 30 years.

The perinatal mortality rate has fallen steadily since the second world war. When comparing data from different countries, rates are falling in most of them at about the same rate, though some countries start worse off and stay there. This reflects the influence of socioeconomic factors and patterns of reproduction more than the quality of obstetric facilities. A similar pattern can be seen to a smaller extent in the regions of the United Kingdom.

The three main causes of perinatal mortality in the United Kingdom are low birth weight, hypoxia, and congenital abnormalities. Low birth weight is currently one of the biggest problems in the Western world (see chapters on small for gestational age and preterm labour). Hypoxia is mostly a problem of labour and to some extent is improved by monitoring women at high risk. Congenital abnormalities may be detected at prenatal examination (see the chapter on detection and management of congenital abnormalities) but the real cure of this problem would be to prevent malformations rather than to detect them and then abort the fetus.

Perinatal mortality rates are not a valid measure of obstetric or midwifery performance. In a developed society they are a mixed measure of a country's educational, social, nutritional, and public health systems as well as of obstetric acute medicine. Probably only a third of the improvement in perinatal mortality statistics is due to improvements in medicine and midwifery. The rest is due to social and economic factors.

Maternal mortality

Maternal deaths are rare in the Western world but this is not so everywhere: in some parts of Africa a woman has a chance as high as one in 25 of dying during one of her pregnancies.

Maternal death usually refers to a woman dying in pregnancy, childbirth, or within 42 days of the end of pregnancy. In many countries, including the United Kingdom, it includes deaths after an abortion or an ectopic pregnancy but in some countries it does not. The definition in Britain used to include deaths up to one year but recently it has come in line with World Health Organisation recommendations.

$$\text{Maternal death rate} = \frac{\begin{array}{c}\text{Deaths in pregnancy, childbirth,}\\ \text{and 6 weeks afterwards} \times 1000\end{array}}{\text{Total maternities}}$$

Maternal death rates in the United Kingdom did not reduce in this century as swiftly as did the rates of perinatal death. Until the mid-1930s maternal mortality was the same as it had been in Victorian times. With the development of chemotherapy and antibiotics the rates reduced; to this was added the improvements brought by a proper blood transfusion service catalysed by the second world war. The founding of the colleges of midwives and obstetricians organised professional training and standards, and the unification of the antenatal and delivery services in the new NHS helped further.

As the maternal death rate is so low, it is hard to see the continued improvement but when the data are plotted on a log scale reduction is still obvious.

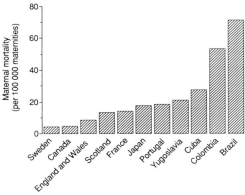

Maternal mortality in various countries
(excluding deaths from abortion)

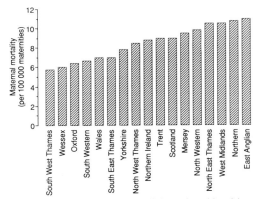

Maternal mortality in the English regional health
authorities and in Wales, Scotland, and Northern
Ireland, 1976-87. Compare the ranking order for
perinatal mortality rate (p 78).

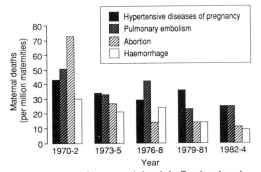

Major causes of maternal death in England and
Wales, 1970-84.

International statistics on maternal mortality are less easy to determine in a comparable way as different countries have different exclusions. In general, however, maternal mortality is an index of medical and midwifery care more than are the perinatal mortality rates. Maternal death rates by region and by country within the United Kingdom also vary but differently from perinatal mortality rates.

In Britain the Confidential Enquiry into Maternal Deaths has been set up to provide information about maternal deaths. A complete case history of each maternal death is obtained and published triennially by the Department of Health, keeping all information confidential. From now on the reports are to be published from the whole United Kingdom rather than separately for the four kingdoms.

The maternal mortality in the United Kingdom was reported to be 7·6 per 100 000 in 1985-7; principal causes of maternal death in England and Wales are hypertension and pulmonary embolism. To reduce the toll of hypertension the inquiry committee recommends that in each region there should be one or two hospitals with staff skilled at looking after pregnant hypertensive mothers and their fetuses. Women with severe degrees of this condition should be electively transferred to these centres by the in-utero transfer service. Pulmonary embolism commonly follows popliteal or pelvic vein thrombosis, which should be watched for, particularly in the puerperium after an operative delivery. An active policy of anticoagulation on suspicion could reduce this cause of death.

Other major killers in the past were infection and haemorrhage; currently these are much reduced. It must give satisfaction to those who fought for the Abortion Act of 1967 to find that in the last two triennia reported by the confidential inquiry committee (1982-4 and 1985-7) there was not a single death from illegal abortion in England and Wales.

Conclusions

Too many doctors think of vital statistics in terms of Disraeli's, "Lies, damn lies and statistics."

Perhaps they should look at statistics in the same way as did Richard Asher:

"When something can be expressed in a numerical way, it is an aid to more precise and accurate thinking."[1]

Most of the data on death rates in England and Wales are derived from the Office of Population Censuses and Surveys. The data on maternal mortality come from the Confidential Inquiries into Maternal Deaths.

1 Holland R, ed. *A sense of Asher.* London: British Medical Association, 1984.

Recommended reading

Barron SL, Macfarlane AJ. Collection and use of routine maternity data. *Baillieres Clin Obstet Gynaecol* 1990;4:681-97.
Macfarlane A, Mugford M. *Birth counts.* London: HMSO, 1984.
Abrams ME, Metters JS. *Confidential enquiries into maternal deaths in England and Wales 1985-1987.* London: HMSO, 1991.

L'ENVOI

The development of antenatal care reflects what has happened in all of medicine—first came the clinical observations, then the intervention of a lot of investigations, each followed by a scientific pedigree, and only later a guilty sideways look at what value it all provides. In an ideal world all the investigations would have been subjected to rigorous scrutiny—randomised controlled trials and careful checks of sensitivity and specificity. Such intellectual disciplines were introduced after many of the tests had been started, but the future of antenatal care depends on deciding which investigations are really useful, applying them more widely, and putting the less helpful ones aside. If we were to make proper use of the proved valuable tests we already have, much effort and money would be saved; we could spend more time listening to and talking with the women we care for. The golden age of antenatal care would have arrived.

GC

INDEX

Abdomen
  circumference, fetal   16, 61, 64
  decompression   64
  distension   46
  examination   11, 12
  surgery   34, 49
Abdominal pain   54
  diagnosis   46
  extrapelvic causes   48-49
  extraperitoneal causes   50
  pelvic causes   31, 33, 34, 46-48, 49, 57
  source   46
Abortion
  criminal   33, 79
  missed   32, 33
  recurrent   32, 33
  septic   31, 33
  therapeutic   32
  See also Miscarriage
Abortion Act 1967   21, 79
Acetylcholinesterase   23
Acidaemia   44
Acidosis, fetal   18
Adrenal gland   8
Adrenaline   8
Adrenocorticotrophic hormone   7, 8
Africa   78
Agriculture   29
Aims of antenatal care   9
Albuminuria   45
Alcohol intake   10, 62-63
Altitude   63
Amniocentesis   24-25
  risk of miscarriage   22, 25, 72
Amniotic fluid
  embolus   57
  volume   13, 17, 24
Ampicillin   45
Anaemia   11, 35
  causes   42
  folate deficiency   43
  haemolytic anaemia   44
  haemorrhagic   44
  iron deficiency   43
  multiple pregnancy   72
  pernicious   43
  sickle cell   44
  thalassaemia   44
Analgesia   47, 48
Anencephaly   23, 25, 62
Angiotensin I   8
Angiotensin II   51
Animal workers   29
Anorexia   49
Antenatal clinics   1, 2
  education   14
Antenatal visits   9
  booking   10-12
  subsequent   12-13
  twins   74
Antepartum haemorrhage   67
  fetal origin   60
  general causes   59
  lower genital tract   59
  perinatal mortality   60
  placenta praevia   58-59
  placental abruption   56-58
  twin pregnancy   72
  unknown origin   60

Antibiotics   33, 44, 45, 48, 68
Anticoagulants   38, 79
Anticonvulsants   40
Antihypertensive drugs   53
Antithyroid drugs   40
Aorta   5
  coarctation   38
Appendicitis   34, 67
  signs and symptoms   49
Appendicectomy   49
Arcuate arteries   19
Aspirin   42, 44, 52, 53, 64
Atenolol   53
Atrial septal defects   38
Azathioprine   63

Bacteriuria   12, 48
  asymptomatic   45
Bed rest   33, 47, 48, 50, 64
  hypertension   52, 72
β Blockers   53
β Mimetics   64, 69
Biological hazards   29
Biparietal diameter   12, 16, 17, 73
Birth rates   76
Birth weight   15
  alcohol intake   63
  effect of work   29, 30
  gestational age   61-62
  maternal influence   63
  multiple pregnancy   73
  paternal influence   63
  perinatal mortality   66
  smoking   62, 63, 65
Bladder   7, 45
Blood
  clotting   57, 58
  dysplasia   36
  film   42, 43, 44
  glucose   39, 40
  investigations   11-12
  volume   6, 72
Blood flow
  changes in pregnancy   8, 29
  Doppler studies   19, 52, 64
Blood pressure   6, 11, 12, 74
  measurement   52
  See also Hypertension
Blood transfusion   43, 58, 59
  exchange   44
  packed red cell   44
Bone marrow   43
Booking visit
  examination   11
  history   10-11
  investigations   11-12
Boredom   29
Bradycardia, fetal   18
Breast milk   7, 28
Breasts   3
Breathing   6
Breech presentation   13,59

Caesarean section   39, 45, 58, 59, 60, 72
  hypertension   53, 55
Calcium antagonists   69
Campbell, Janet   1
Carbamazepine   63
Cardiac failure   37

Cardiac output   5, 37
Cardiomyopathy   37
Cardiotocography   18, 52
Cardiovascular system   5-6, 37
Carotoid arteries, fetal   19
Central nervous system abnormalities   23, 25
Central venous pressure   33, 58
Cerebral oedema   54
Cervix
  assessment   13, 49, 73, 74
  benign lesions   36, 59
  changes   3, 8
  carcinoma   36, 59
  cerclage   67, 73
  incompetence   32, 67
  pain   34
  smear test   11
Chemical hazards   28
Chest infections   44
Chest radiography   6, 12
Chlamydia, ovine   29
Cholecystitis   49
Cholestasis   41
Chorioamnionitis   67
Choriocarcinoma   35
Chorionic villus sampling   16
  abortion rates   22
  advantages   22
  technique   22
Chromosomal abnormalities   32, 62
  diagnosis   21, 22, 24-25, 26
Clearview pregnancy test   4
Cleft palate   19
Clonidine   53
Coagulases   67
Coagulopathy   33, 52, 57
Colic   49
Complement system   52
Confidential Enquiries into Maternal Deaths   53, 79
Congenital abnormalities   12, 39, 40, 62
  availability of tests   25-26
  causes   21
  chromosomal   22, 24-25, 26, 62
  multiple pregnancy   72
  reasons for diagnosis   21
  structural   23-24, 25
Congenital heart disease
  fetal   38, 72
  maternal   37, 38
Convulsions See Eclampsia
Cordocentesis   19, 25
Cortisol   7, 8
Creatinine   7
Crown-rump length   16
Cyclo-oxygenase   52, 53
Cystic fibrosis   21
Cytomegalovirus   12, 32, 62

Decidua   31, 32, 33
Delivery
  diabetic mothers   39
  expected date   10
  hypertension and eclampsia   54-55
  intrauterine growth retardation   65
  location   2
  preterm labour   70
Dental care   11
Deoxycorticosterone   8

Index

Dermoid cyst 48
Diabetes 33, 69
  delivery 39
  gestational 40
  incidence 38
  insulin dependent 39
  non-insulin dependent 39, 40
Diaphragm 6
Diazepam 40, 54
Diet 10, 40
  folate rich 43
  high fibre 42
  iron rich 42, 43
Disseminated intravascular coagulopathy 33, 57
Diuretics 52
DNA 22, 24, 26, 43
Doppler ultrasonography 19, 52, 60, 64, 65
Down's syndrome *See* Trisomy 21
Duodenal atresia 24, 62
Dwarfism 12
Dysuria 45

Echocardiography 6
Eclampsia 51, 72
  delivery 55
  imminent 54
  maternal death 54
  treatment 54
Ectopic pregnancy 33, 47
  causes 34
  management 34-35
  presentation 34
  recurrence 34, 35
  sites 34
Education 14
  preterm delivery 68
Eisenmenger's syndrome 38
Elastases 67
Electrocardiogram 6
ELISA 4
Embryonic sac 15
Endocarditis 38
Endocrine system 7-8
  imbalance 33
Environment
  congenital abnormalities 21
  working 29
Enzyme linked immunosorbent assay 4
Epidural anaesthesia 54
Epilepsy 40
Escherichia coli 31
European Community 77
Examination at booking visit 11
Exercise 29
Expiratory volume 6

Fallopian tubes
  removal 34, 35
  torsion 47
Family history 10
Family size, completed 76
Fatigue 29
Femur length 17, 26
Ferritin 42
Ferrous fumarate 43
Ferrous succinate 43
Ferrous sulphate 43
Fetal alcohol syndrome 63
Fetal brain 24
  damage 64
Fetal death 23, 44, 56
  cordocentesis 19
Fetal growth 11, 12
  measurements 16-17
  See also Intrauterine growth retardation
Fetal head
  biparietal diameter 12, 16, 17
  circumference 64
Fetal heart 12, 13, 23, 74
  pulse 15
  rate 18, 52, 60, 64
Fetal measurement laboratory 65
Fetocide 72
α Fetoprotein 22, 23, 25

Fetoscopy 19
Fetus
  abdominal circumference 16, 61, 64
  blood flow 19, 54-55
  blood loss 19
  blood sampling 19
  hypoxia 53, 60, 78
  lie and presentation 12, 74
  metabolism 17
  movements 18
  oxygen consumption 5
  weight 17, 61, 64, 73
Fever 31, 45, 47, 48
Fibrinogen 57
Fibroids 47
  red degeneration 47, 57
Fits, eclamptic 54
Fluids
  intake 45, 48
  intravenous 33, 44, 47, 58
Folate
  absorption 40
  deficiency anaemia 43, 72
  foods 43
  sickle cell disease 44
  supplements 10, 72
Folic acid 40, 43
Folinic acid 36
Follicle stimulating hormone 3, 7

Gall stones 41
Gastroschisis 23, 62
General fertility rate 76
General practitioners 2, 3, 9
Genetic abnormalities *See* Chromosomal
  abnormalities
Genital tract 8
German measles *See* Rubella
Gestation calculator 10
Gestational diabetes 40
Gestational length
  birth weight 61, 62
  long 13
  multiple pregnancy 67, 73
  neonatal mortality 66
Gestational trophoblastic disease
  causes 35
  management 36
  presentation 35
Glomerular filtration rate 7
Glycosuria 12, 38, 40
Glucose, blood 39, 40
Glucose tolerance tests 40
Glycogen 16
Goitre, fetal 40
Gonadotrophins 3, 7
Gravidity 11
Growth hormone 7

Haematological values 42
Haematoma
  rectus 50
  round ligament 48
Haemodilution 6
Haemoglobin concentrations 42, 43, 44
Haemoglobins C and S 44
Haemoglobinopathies 44
Haemolysis 42, 44
Haemorrhage 79
  See also Antepartum haemorrhage; Vaginal
  bleeding
Haemorrhagic anaemia 44
Hare lip 19
Headache 54
Health and Safety Executive 28, 29
Heart 5, 6, 11
  sounds
  See also Fetal heart
Heart disease 69
  causes 37-38
  congenital 37, 38, 72
  management 38
  rheumatic 37
  risk to fetus 38

Heart valves 6
  artificial 38
Heat, local 45, 48
Height 11
Heparin 38
Hepatitis 12, 41
Historical background 1
HIV 12
HLA antigens 32
Hodgkin's disease 59
Home deliveries 2
Hookworms 42, 44
Hormone tests 19, 64
  miscarriage 16
Hospital antenatal clinics 1, 2
Housework 28
Human chorionic gonadotrophin 16, 22
  hydatidiform mole 35, 36
  pregnancy tests 3
Human Fertilisation and Embryology
  Authority 71
Human placental lactogen 7, 19
Hydatidiform mole 35
  management 36
Hydralazine 53, 54
Hydrocephalus 24
Hydronephrosis 24
Hypertension 32, 35, 39
  categories and definitions 51
  causes 51
  delivery 54-55
  detection 52
  eclampsia 54
  intrauterine growth retardation 52, 55, 63
  management 52-53
  maternal death 79
  multiple pregnancy 72
  pain 50
  prediction 19
  proteinuria 51, 52, 54
Hyperthyroidism 8, 33, 40, 69
Hypothalamus 7
Hypothyroidism 40
Hypovolaemia 46
Hypoxaemia 18
Hypoxia 44
  fetal 53, 60, 78
Hysterogram 32

IgG antibodies 40
Immunological rejection
  fetus 32
  transplant recipients 45
In utero transfer 65, 70
Induction of labour 13, 40, 53, 55
  preterm 68
Industry 29
Infant death 77
Infections 32, 39, 79
  chest 44
  intrauterine 62, 67
  membranes 67
  urinary tract 7, 44, 45, 48
  vaginal 36, 68
Inspiratory volume 6
Insulin 39
Intensive care units 53, 55
Interim Licensing Authority 71
Intestines
  blood supply 29
  fetal 24
  x rays 28
Intrauterine growth retardation
  causes 44, 52, 55, 62-63
  diagnosis 63-64
  multiple pregnancy 73
  treatment 64-65
Intrauterine infection 62, 67
Intravenous hydration 33, 44, 47, 58
Investigations, initial 11-12
Iodine 8, 40
Iron
  absorption 42
  intake 42

parenteral 43
tablets 43
Iron deficiency anaemia 44
folate deficiency 43
indices 42
prevention 42
treatment 43
Itching, facial 54

Jaundice 40

Kick chart 18
Kidneys 7, 52
blood supply 29
damage 52
disease 32, 45
fetal abnormalities 12, 24
necrosis 58
Klinefelter's syndrome 72
Kyphosis 11

Labetalol 53
Labour 7, 8
induction 13, 40, 53, 55, 68
long 40
See also Preterm labour
Laparoscopy 35, 46, 47
scars 11
Laparotomy 47, 48, 49, 50
Legs 11, 29
Leucocytes, fetal 19, 25
Leukaemia 36, 59
Ligaments, pelvic 8, 48
Limb malformations 21, 23
Listeriosis 32
Liver 41
fetal 16
oedema 50, 54
Lungs 6, 11
Luteinising hormone 3, 7

Macrosomia 40, 69
Magnesium sulphate 54
Malaria 62
Malnutrition 32, 42
Maternal age 22, 27, 71
Maternal death rate 78
Maternal deaths 44
Confidential Enquiries 53, 79
definition 78
eclampsia 54
United Kingdom 78, 79
Maternity leave 27
Maternity payments 27
Medical history 10, 67
Megaloblastic anaemia 43, 72
Membrane rupture, premature 67
Meningocele 23
Menstrual history 10
Methadone 63
Methotrexate 36
Methyldopa 53
Microcephaly 12
Micturition frequency 7, 45
Midwives 2, 9
Mines Act 1889 28
Miscarriage 46
amniocentesis 22, 25, 72
causes 32-33
chorionic villus sampling 22
complete 31, 33
hormone tests 16
incomplete 31
inevitable 31, 33
management 33
presentation 33
recurrent 32
threatened 31, 33
visual display units (VDU) 29
Mitral stenosis 37
Monilia 36, 59
Morphine 58
Multigravidas 9
Multiple pregnancy 23

diagnosis 71
management 74
outcome 75
preterm labour 67, 73
prevalence 71
problems 72-73
types 71
Myometrial cells 8

Narcotics 63
National Birthday Trust, British Births
Survey 61
National Perinatal Epidemiological Unit,
Oxford 1
Nausea 46, 49, 72
Neonatal death rate 77
gestational age at birth 66
socioeconomic class 10
Neonatal thyrotoxicosis 40
Netherlands 9
Neural tube defects 23, 25, 40, 72
Neutrophils 43
Nitrofurantoin 45
Noradrenaline 8
Nutrition 62
fetal 16

Obesity 40, 62
Obstetric history 11, 67
Oedema 11, 52
cerebral 54
liver 50, 54
pulmonary 37, 69
Oestriol 19, 22, 64
Oestrogens 7, 8, 64
Office of Population Censuses and Surveys 76
Oligohydramnios 17, 63, 64
Oliguria 58
Omphalocele 12, 62
Osteogenesis imperfecta 62
Ovarian arteries 8
Ovaries
torsion 47
tumours 34, 48, 67
Oxygen consumption 5
Oxytocic agents 33
Oxytocin 7, 36

Parity 11
Pelvic arthropathy 50
Pelvis, bony 11, 13
Peptic ulceration 44
Perinatal mortality 13, 44, 65
amniotic fluid volume 17
antepartum haemorrhage 60
birth weight 66
causes 78
falling rates 78
maternal factors 15
multiple pregnancy 75
rate 77
Peripheral resistance 6
Peritonitis 49
Pernicious anaemia 43
Pfannenstiel's scars 11
Phenytoin 40, 54
Physical hazards 28-29
Piles 44
Pituitary gland 7
hormones 3, 7
Placenta 24
bleeding 23, 56, 60
hormones 8
insufficiency 16, 64
vascular resistance 52
water transfer 7
Placenta praevia 57, 72
aim of treatment 59
diagnosis 59
grades 58
vaginal examination 59
Placental abruption 46, 49, 72
cause 57
concealed 56

diagnosis 57
management 58
pathology 57
revealed 56
Placental bed
blood supply 8, 19, 64
vessel spasm 56, 57
Plasma expanders 58
Plasma volume 6
Platelet
aggregation 51, 53
count 52
enzymes 52, 53
Polyhydramnios 57, 67, 73
Population 77
Postneonatal death 77
Potassium chloride 72
Potassium citrate 45
Potter's syndrome 62
Pouch of Douglas 34, 35
Pre-eclampsia 41, 44, 51
symptoms and signs 54
Pregnancy
diagnostic tests 3-4
end 13
energy requirements 62
termination 21, 32
signs and symptoms 3
Prepregnancy care 10
Preterm labour 49
causes 66-68
defining 66
delivery 70
diagnosis 68
effect of work 29
inhibition 69
multiple pregnancy 73
prevention 68
Primigravidas 11
antenatal visits 9
Progesterone 6, 7, 11, 19
miscarriage 33, 48
Progestogens 33, 48
Prolactin 7
Propranolol 53
Prostacyclin 51
Prostaglandin pessaries 55
Prostaglandin synthesis inhibitors 69
Prostaglandins 67
Proteases 67
Proteinuria 12, 74
hypertension 51, 52, 54
Pulmonary embolism 79
Pulmonary hypertension 38
Pulmonary oedema 37, 69
Pulse
fetal heart 15
pressure 6
rate 5
Pyelonephritis 45, 48, 67

Quadruplets 71, 73, 75

Radiography 6, 12
safety 28-29
Radioisotopes 29
Rectal examination 49
Rectus haematoma 50
Red cells 6, 42
life 44
transfusion 44
Reflex responses 54
Regional centres
hypertension 53, 55
investigations 20
Relaxin 50
Renal arteries, fetal 19
Renal blood flow 7
Renin 8
Respiratory distress syndrome 65
Respiratory system 6
Reticulocytes 42
Retinopathy, diabetic 39
Rheumatic heart disease 37

Index

Ribs 6
Ritodrine 69, 73
Rubella 10, 12, 29, 32
  congenital 62

Salbutamol 69
Salpingitis 33
Salpingostomy 35
Schwangerschaftsprotein 1 16
Scoliosis 11
Scottish twin survey 71, 72
Sedatives 52
Septic abortion 31
  management 33
Sex determination 23
Sexual intercourse 33, 73
Shock 46, 57, 58, 59
  endotoxic 31
Shoe size 11
Shoulder dystocia 40
Sickle cell crisis 44
Sickle cell disease 44
Skeletal dysplasia 17
Small for gestational age
  causes 62-63
  defining 61-62
  delivery 65
  diagnosis 63-64
  treatment 64-65
Smoking 10
  birth weight 62, 63, 65
Social benefits 14
Sociobiological background 10, 15, 66
Sodium chloride test 44
Sodium nitroprusside 53
Spina bifida 12, 23, 25
Spinal cord degeneration 43
Spine 11
Spiral arteries 54
  atherosis 52
  trophoblastic invasion 51
Status epilepticus 40
Steroids 41, 69
Stillbirth rates 77
  socioeconomic class 10
Streptococci, β haemolytic 67
Streptococcus faecalis 31
Stress 29, 30
Stroke 53
Switzerland 9
Sympathomimetics *See* β mimetics
Symphysiofundal height 12, 13, 73, 74
Symphysis pubis 50
Syphilis 12, 62

Tapeworms 44
Teeth 11
  extraction 38
Teratogenesis 28, 38, 40
Tetralogy of Fallot 38

Thalassaemia 44
Thrombosis 10, 79
Thromboxane 51, 53
Thyroid crisis 40
Thyroid disease 40
Thyroid gland 8, 11
  surgery 40
Thyrotoxicosis 40
Thyrotrophin 7
Thyroxine 8
Tocography 68
Tocolytic agents 68, 69
Toxoplasmosis 12, 32, 62
Transplant recipients 45
Transverse lie 59
Travel 30
Trimethoprim 45
Triplets 71, 73, 75
Trisomy 21 (Down's syndrome) 62
  amniocentesis 25
  biochemical screening 22, 26
  cost of diagnosis 26
  risk 22
Trophoblastic invasion 51
Tubal ectopic pregnancy
  leaking 34, 35
  rupture 34
Turner's syndrome 72
Twin pregnancy 57, 67
  diagnosis 71
  hospital admission 74
  lie and presentation 74
  management 74
  mechanisms 71
  outcome 75
  preterm labour 73
  prevalence 71
  problems 72-73

Ulcerative colitis 10
Ultrasonography 11, 12, 32, 35, 39, 46, 57, 58, 59
  Doppler 19, 52, 60, 64
  early pregnancy 15
  fetal abnormalities 23-24, 25
  fetal growth 16-17, 65
  intrauterine growth retardation 63-64
  multiple pregnancy 71, 74
  safety 29
Umbilical arteries 19, 55
Uptake of care 1
Urea 7
Ureters 7, 45
Urethral stretch 47
Urinary system 7
Urinary tract
  abnormalities 45, 48
  infection 7, 44, 45, 48
  lithiasis 49
Urine

alkalination 45
  fetal 17
  output 33, 58
  retention 47
  tests 12
Urography 28, 45
Uterine blood flow 8
  Doppler studies 19, 64
  exercise 29
  improving 64
Uterus
  abnormalities 32, 57, 67
  changes 3, 8, 11, 12
  contractions 49, 68
  infection 62, 67
  retroverted 47
  rupture 57

Vaginal bleeding
  causes 31
  ectopic pregnancy 34-35
  gestational trophoblastic disease 35-36
  local causes 36
  maternal disease 36
  miscarriage 31-33
  See also Antepartum haemorrhage
Vaginal examination 11, 13, 34
  placenta praevia 59
Vaginal infection 36, 68
Valproates 63
Varicose veins 11, 59, 72
Vasa praevia 60
Visits *See* Antenatal visits
Visual display units 29
Visual disturbances 54
Vitamin deficiencies 32, 43
Vitamin K 40
Volvulus 49
Vomiting 35, 46, 47, 50
  pain 48
von Willebrand's disease 36, 59

Warfarin 38
Weight 11, 12
  fetal 17, 61, 64, 73
  See also Birth weight
Work in pregnancy
  biological hazards 29
  birth weight 29, 30
  chemical hazards 28
  environment 29
  maternity leave 27
  physical hazards 28-29
  strenuous 29
  travel 30
Working women 27
  types of work 28

x ray safety 28-29